CAMBRIDGE LIBRARY COLLECTION

Books of enduring scholarly value

History of Medicine

It is sobering to realise that as recently as the year in which *On the Origin of Species* was published, learned opinion was that diseases such as typhus and cholera were spread by a 'miasma', and suggestions that doctors should wash their hands before examining patients were greeted with mockery by the profession. The Cambridge Library Collection reissues milestone publications in the history of Western medicine as well as studies of other medical traditions. Its coverage ranges from Galen on anatomical procedures to Florence Nightingale's common-sense advice to nurses, and includes early research into genetics and mental health, colonial reports on tropical diseases, documents on public health and military medicine, and publications on spa culture and medicinal plants.

The Works of John Hunter, F.R.S.

The surgeon and anatomist John Hunter (1728–93) left a famous legacy in the Hunterian Museum of medical specimens now in the Royal College of Surgeons, and in this collection of his writings, edited by James Palmer, with a biography by Drewry Ottley, published between 1835 and 1837. The first four volumes are of text, and the larger Volume 5 contains plates. Hunter had begun his career as a demonstrator in the anatomy classes of his brother William, before qualifying as a surgeon. He regarded surgery as evidence of failure – the mutilation of a patient who could not be cured by other means – and his studies of anatomy and natural history were driven by his belief that it was necessary to understand the normal physiological processes before attempting to cure the abnormal ones. Volume 5 contains the plates which accompany the works in the other volumes, with notes.

The Works of
John Hunter, F.R.S.

VOLUME 5: PLATES

EDITED BY JAMES F. PALMER

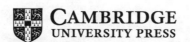

CAMBRIDGE
UNIVERSITY PRESS

University Printing House, Cambridge, CB2 8BS, United Kingdom

Cambridge University Press is part of the University of Cambridge.

It furthers the University's mission by disseminating knowledge in the pursuit of
education, learning and research at the highest international levels of excellence.

www.cambridge.org
Information on this title: www.cambridge.org/9781108079617

© in this compilation Cambridge University Press 2015

This edition first published 1837
This digitally printed version 2015

ISBN 978-1-108-07961-7 Paperback

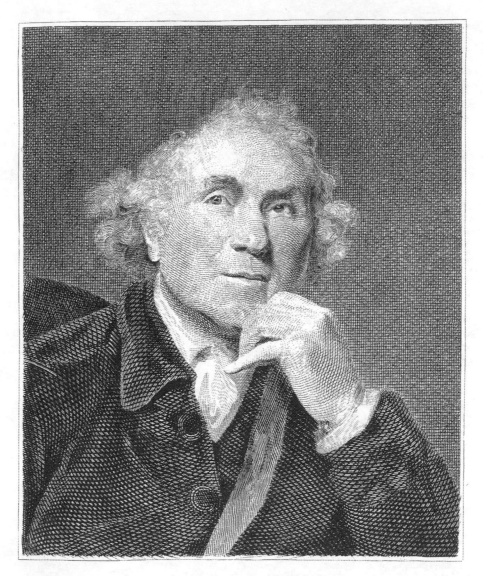

Reynolds Pinx.   London, Published Jan. 1. 1788, by W. Sharp.   Sharp Sculp

THE

WORKS

OF

JOHN HUNTER, F.R.S.

WITH

NOTES.

EDITED BY

JAMES F. PALMER,

SENIOR SURGEON TO THE ST. GEORGE'S AND ST. JAMES'S DISPENSARY; FELLOW OF THE ROYAL
MEDICAL AND CHIRURGICAL SOCIETY OF LONDON, ETC.

———————

PLATES.

———————

LONDON:

PUBLISHED BY

LONGMAN, REES, ORME, BROWN, GREEN, AND LONGMAN,
PATERNOSTER-ROW.
1837.

PRINTED BY RICHARD TAYLOR,
RED LION COURT, FLEET STREET.

EXPLANATION OF PLATES.

PLATE I.

Fig. 1. A representation of the under-side of the upper-jaw, without the teeth. *a a a a a* the outer line of the circle, or what is commonly called the outer plate of the alveolar process. *b b b* the inner line of the circle, commonly called the inner plate.' *c c* the ten single sockets, viz. for the incisores, cuspidati, and bicuspides. *d d* the three double sockets for the molary, or triple-fanged teeth ; the two first having three sockets, and the last only two.

Fig. 2. A representation of the upper-part of the lower-jaw, showing particularly the sockets of the teeth. *a* the sockets of the ten single-fanged teeth. *b* the sockets of the three double-fanged teeth.

Fig. 3. A sketch of the joint and muscles of the lower-jaw to explain what was said of its motions. *a* the condyle of the lower-jaw. *b* the angle of the lower-jaw. *c* the moveable cartilage of the joint. *d* the eminence before the cavity, or hollow in the temporal bone for the articulation of the lower-jaw. *e* the cavity itself. *f* the meatus auditorius externus. *g* the origin of the digastric muscle. *h* one of the vertebræ of the neck. *i* the last molar tooth. *j* the insertion of the digastric muscle.

PLATE II.

Fig. 1. A front view of the upper- and lower-jaws of an adult, with a full set of teeth. *a a a* the upper-jaw. *b b* the lower-jaw.

Fig. 2. A side view of both jaws in the same state. *a a* the upper-jaw. *b b* the lower-jaw. *c* its ascending process. *d* the root of the coronoid process. *e* the condyle. *f f f f* the fluted alveolar processes.

PLATE III.

Fig. 1. The basis of the upper-jaw, with a full set of teeth, showing the cutting edges and grinding surfaces of the teeth of the upper-jaw. *a a a a* the four incisores. *b b* the two cuspidati. *c c* the four bicuspides. *d d* the six grinders.

Fig. 2. A view from above and behind of the lower-jaw, with a full set of teeth ; showing the cutting edges and grinding surfaces of the teeth of that jaw, with the coronoid processes, and condyles for articulation. *a a a a* the four incisores. *b b* the two cuspidati. *c c* the four bicuspides. *d d* the six grinders. *e e* the coronoid processes. *f f* the condyles.

Fig. 3. The moveable cartilage of the joint of the lower-jaw. *a* the cut surface of a longitudinal section of it : the lower and concave surface is what is articulated with the condyle, the upper and convex surface is what is in contact with the temporal bone.

Fig. 4. A side view of the upper- and lower-jaw, in which the outer plate of the alveolar process was

A 2

taken off to expose the fangs of the teeth in their sockets. The length of each fang is at once seen with respect to its neighbour, and this kind of articulation pointed out at one view.

PLATE IV.

The bones of the face and part of the head of a very old woman, who had lost her teeth a considerable time before death. The whole alveolar processes are gone in both jaws, which allows of the lower-jaw being raised above two inches higher than what is common in shutting the mouth, before the gums of both jaws can come into contact. By this increased motion of the lower-jaw, the chin is brought more upon a line with the articulation, and therefore projects beyond the upper-jaw considerably.

PLATE V.

Fig. 1. Two views of the sixteen teeth of one side of both jaws, taken out of their sockets to expose the whole of each tooth.

Row 1. The teeth of the upper-jaw, seen from the outside.

Row 2. The same view of the teeth of the lower-jaw : the five single are similar to those of the upper-jaw, but the grinders in this have only two fangs. *a* the incisors. *b* the cuspidati. *c c* the bicuspides. *d d* the two first grinders, having three fangs. *e* the third grinder, or dens sapientiæ, having also three fangs.

Row 3 & 4. A side view of the same teeth, showing that the incisores and cuspidati, in this view, differ from the former view more than the bicuspides or grinders.

Row 3. *a a* the two incisores of the upper-jaw, showing the hollowed inner surface of the body of these teeth. *b* the cuspidatus, showing the same. *c c* the bicuspides, showing the two points at the basis of each. The first of them has a forked fang.

Fig. 1—7. Show the cavities of the teeth in the incisores, cuspidatus, bicuspidatus and molares.

Fig. 8. A molaris of the lower-jaw, with part of its fangs sawed off, to show that the sides of the cavity or canal have grown together, and divided it into two small canals, which are represented by the four dark points.

Fig. 9—10. The cavity in the body of the teeth seen in transverse sections.

Fig. 11—12. Longitudinal sections of the molares to expose the cavities.

Fig. 13. The basis of a molaris whose points were worn down, and the bony part which projected into those points exposed.

Fig. 14. A molaris whose bony part is wholly exposed, and only a circle of enamel left, covering the sides all round.

Fig. 15—16. A lateral view of the enamel of a molaris and bicuspis, cut longitudinally.

Fig. 17. A cuspidatus worn so much down as to expose the whole end of the bony part, a circle only of enamel remaining.

Fig. 18. An incisor slit down its axis, to show the enamel upon the body of the tooth, covering much more of the convex than of the concave part.

Fig. 19. An incisor, showing the same as fig 17.

Fig. 20. A horse's tooth slit down its whole length, to show how the enamel is intermixed with the bony part, and that it passes through the whole length of the tooth. The enamel is represented by the white lines, which are penniform, showing the striated texture of the enamel.

Fig. 21. The grinding surface of a horse's molaris, to show the irregular course of the enamel.

Fig. 22. An incisor a little magnified, slit down its middle, to show that the enamel is striated, and that the striæ are turned towards the centre.

Fig. 23. A grinder in the same state, to show the same circumstances.

Fig. 24. The basis of a molaris broken through, showing that the enamel is striated in this view also, and that the striæ point to the centre. N.B. The teeth must be broken to show these facts.

Fig. 25. An old tooth, whose basis has been worn down below the original termination of the cavity in the body of the tooth, and that end has been filled up, in the same proportion with new matter, to prevent the cavity being exposed. This matter is of a darker colour, as represented in the figure.

Fig. 26. Another tooth in the same state.

PLATE VI.

Fig. 1—10. Show the gradual growth of the two jaws, especially of the alveolar processes.

Fig. 1—2. One side of the lower and of the upper-jaw of a fœtus, about three or four months old. *a a* the groove which is afterwards formed into sockets.

Fig. 3—4. One side of the lower- and of the upper-jaw of a fœtus about six months old, at which age some of the partitions *a a* have shot across near the anterior part, forming distinct cells.

Fig. 5—6. The upper- and lower-joint of a new-born child, showing the last-mentioned circumstance in a more advanced state.

Fig. 7. The lower-jaw of a child seven or eight months old, (in which the two first incisors had cut the gum,) showing the sockets of six teeth. The mouths of the alveoli are observed to be contracted over the teeth, especially those of the grinders, where they have not yet begun to open for the passage of the teeth.

Fig. 8. A sketch of an upper-jaw, where the cuspidatus of that side had been formed high up in the jaw, and therefore never could appear through the gum. *a* the fang of the cuspidatus. *b* its body contained in the upper-jaw and alveolar process.

Fig. 9. A sketch of the upper-jaw of a child, where the cuspidatus was inverted, so that its point was turned up against the jaw, and the growing mouth of its cavity towards the gum. *a* the point of the cuspidatus turned up against the jaw. *b* the open and growing part of the tooth, which should be formed into a fang.

Fig. 10. The outline of the lower-jaw of a child, to show that the condyle is then nearly on a line with the gums.

Fig. 11. One side of the upper- and lower-jaw of a subject about eight or nine years of age, where the incisores and cuspidati of the fœtus were shed, and their successors rising in new sockets; showing likewise the two grinders of the child, with the bicuspides forming underneath. The adult grinder was ready to cut the gum; and the second grinder of the lower-jaw is lodged in the root of the coronoid process, and in the upper-jaw it is in the tubercle.

Fig. 12. Part of the lower-jaw cut through at the symphysis. The incisor of the child is standing in its socket, and the adult incisor forming in a distinct socket underneath.

Fig. 13. Another view of the same piece of the jaw, to show that the bicuspides are formed in distinct sockets of their own, and not in the socket of the grinder which stands above.

6 EXPLANATION OF PLATES.

PLATE VII.

Fig. 1. The five teeth in the half of each jaw of a fœtus of seven or eight months, showing the progress of ossification from the first incisor to the second grinder.

Fig. 2. The same teeth somewhat further advanced.

Fig. 3. The teeth of a child eight or nine years of age, showing the five temporary teeth in a more advanced state, with the first adult grinder. The adult incisores and one cuspidatus are also begun to be formed.

Fig. 4. The teeth of one side of both jaws, from a child of five or six years of age. B B, C C the temporary teeth almost completely formed. A D seven; viz., four above and three below, of the succeeding teeth, seen at the roots of the first set. E E the bodies of the first adult grinders nearly formed.

Fig. 5. The teeth of one side of both jaws, from a child of seven years of age. This is an age in which there are more teeth formed and forming than at any other time of life. B C, C C the ten temporary teeth complete. A D ten incomplete to succeed them. E E two adult grinders, making twenty-two in this side, and of course forty-four in the whole. *a a a a* the fangs of the temporary teeth, beginning to decay at their points.

Fig. 6. The teeth of a child eight or nine years old; principally to show the progress of the second set, and the beginning and decay of the first set. A A the first incisores of the second or permanent set. B the second incisor. C the cuspidatus. D E the bicuspides. F G the two first molares. *a b* the temporary incisores, the first of which in the upper-jaw is wanting, having been shed. *c* the cuspidati. *d e* the temporary molares.

Fig. 7. The teeth of a youth about eleven or twelve years old, showing the further progress of the one set towards perfection, and of the other in their decay. *a a a a* the incisores of the second set, which had all cut the gum. *b b* the basis of the third molaris, or dens sapientiæ. *c c* the remaining molares of the first set, with decayed fangs. *d d* the two first molares of the second set, so much advanced that they had cut the gums.

PLATE VIII.

Fig. 1—2. The lower- and upper-jaw of a fœtus, from which part of the gum and bony socket is taken off, to expose the membrane which incloses the teeth.

Fig. 3. The lower-jaw of a new-born child, where this inclosing membrane is opened, to show the bodies of the teeth which were covered by it. The blood-vessels which run in its substance are also exposed.

Fig. 4. That part of the jaw and gum which contains the cuspidatus: the whole is a little magnified. The membrane is opened and turned off on each side, and the fore-part is turned down: the upper part of the pulp is covered with its bony shell, which is seen by its want of vessels.

Fig. 5 and 6. The pulp of a cuspidatus, and the pulp of a grinder, magnified. The ossifications are removed to show that the pulps are of the same shape with the teeth which are formed upon them. As far down on the pulp as the vessels are seen, the ossification had advanced; which shows that it is more vascular where the operation of ossification is going on. The lower ragged edges represent the borders of the capsulæ turned down.

Fig. 7. One of the grinders of the lower-jaw, sawed down to expose the two cavities or canals leading to the body of the tooth, where they unite and form a square cavity. In these two canals are seen two arteries, which run on to the common cavity, and there ramify. The veins are not injected. The whole is magnified. In the body of the tooth may be observed a number of strata, each of which is lost in the circumference of the tooth.

Fig. 8. An incisor prepared and magnified in the same manner, showing the same circumstances in that tooth.

Fig. 9. The production of the permanent rudiment by means of a process given off from the temporary, shown in a lower incisor.

Fig. 10. The rudiments in a more advanced stage; the permanent being now inclosed in its proper socket, though still connected with the temporary.

Fig. 11. The connection between the temporary tooth and the permanent rudiment, as it exists after the former has passed through the gum.

Fig. 12. A view of the lower-jaw, after the whole of the temporary teeth have passed through the gums, showing the relative position of the temporary teeth, and the rudiments of the permanent at this period.

Fig. 13. Shows the formation and cavity of the fangs of the molares. The upper row are those of the lower-jaw, and the lower those of the upper. A A, *a a* is the common cavity in the body of the tooth; which in the second, *a a*, is deeper than in the first. B shows the bony arch thrown over the mouth of the cavity, and dividing that into two openings, which give origin to the two fangs. C D E the progress of these fangs. F a molaris of the upper-jaw, where the mouth of the cavity is a little tucked in, at three different points, from which three ossifications shoot. G shows these ossifications, and the beginning of these fangs. H I K show the gradual growth of these fangs.

Fig. 14. Is a comparative view of the incisors and grinders of the child and adult; for the better understanding of which they are sawed down the middle, showing, in a side view, the gradual increase of these teeth. The uppermost row is of the child, and the lower of the adult. *a b c d* show the gradual growth of the body, fangs and cavity of the incisors of both ages. *e f g* show these circumstances in the grinders.

Fig. 15. 1—7 show the gradual growth of a single tooth, from its formation nearly, to its being almost complete.

Fig. 16. A series of grinders of the child, from their being complete, to their utmost decay. *a* is a grinder of the upper-jaw nearly complete, in which the three fangs are almost formed. *b* has some of its fang absorbed. *c* more. *d* still more. *e* nearly all gone, and *f* the whole of the fangs gone, only the neck and body remaining.

Fig. 17. A series of incisors in the same state. No. 1. a completely formed tooth; 2, the fang somewhat decayed; 3, more so; 4, still more; 5, the fang almost gone; and 6, the whole fang gone, the neck and body only remaining.

Fig. 18. A horse's tooth that was just ready to be shed. The three parts of the tooth, which stand up, inclosed the rising end of the young tooth. This is all that was left of a long tooth.

PLATE IX.

Fig. 1. The penis slit open, showing a stricture in the urethra, about two inches from the glans. The stricture is but slight. A A the cut surface of the corpus spongiosum urethræ. B B the canal of the urethra, in which may be observed the orifices of the lacunæ. C the stricture.

Fig. 2. The penis slit open for about three inches, to show the lacunæ, which become occasionally an obstruction to the passage of the bougie. A A the corpus spongiosum urethræ. B B the internal surface of the canal of the urethra, pointing to the orifice of two of the lacunæ.   C a bristle introduced into a lacuna. D the end of the bougie introduced into the remaining part of the urethra.

PLATE X.

The urethra opened in two different places, one before the stricture, the other behind : the one before is through the body of the penis, the other behind is upon the anterior surface of the membranous part ; and a bougie passes from the one opening to the other. A A the crura penis and bulbous part of the urethra, all blended together by inflammation and suppuration, which has taken place in many parts. B B the prostate gland in a diseased state. C C the cut edges of the bladder. D the urethra behind the stricture, very much enlarged ; irregular on the surface in consequence of ulceration. E E the cut surfaces of the corpora cavernosa penis.   F F the cut surfaces of the corpus spongiosum urethræ. G G a bougie passing from the sound to the unsound part of the urethra. H a small bougie in the new passage.

PLATE XI.

Two canulas for applying caustic to strictures in the urethra.

Fig. 1. A straight silver canula, with the plug projecting beyond the termination of the canula, making a rounded end ; at the other end of the wire is a small port-crayon, in which is represented a piece of caustic.

Fig. 2. A flexible canula, for applying caustic to strictures in the bend of the urethra. The wire with the small port-crayon, is pushed out beyond its end.

Fig. 3. A piece of silver wire, with the plug at the end, to be introduced into the canula, as in figure 1.

PLATE XII.

The bladder and penis of a person who died of a mortification of the bladder in consequence of a stricture and stone in the urethra.   In this plate not only the stricture is represented, but the thickened coats and fasciculated inner surface of the bladder ; as also the small stone, which acted as a valve or plug ; beside which, a canula is introduced from the glans down to the stricture, showing the practicability of destroying it with caustic. A A the bladder, cut open, showing its coats a little thickened, and its inner surface fasciculated. B the body of the penis. C C the corpus spongiosum urethræ, cut open through its whole length, exposing the urethra. D the prostate gland divided. E a silver canula introduced into the urethra, through which the caustic is passed on to the stricture. F points out the stricture, with the stone lying above, so as entirely to prevent the passage of the urine.

PLATE XIII.

An enlarged prostate gland, particularly the valvular process, which has increased inwards, into the bladder, in form of a tumour; in consequence of which the water passed with difficulty, which became the cause of the increased thickness of the bladder. A the prostate gland. B the projecting part passing into the cavity of the bladder. C C a bristle in the urethra, to show it is above this tumour. D the cut edge of the bladder, which shows its increased thickness.

PLATE XIV.

A kidney, the ureter, pelvis, and infundibula of which are very considerably enlarged in consequence of a stricture in the urethra. A the substance of the kidney, which has become very thin. B B the infundibula much enlarged. C the pelvis very much enlarged. D the ureter increased-more than ten times its natural size.

PLATE XV.

The valvular part of the bladder, so increased as to form a considerable tumour, projecting into the cavity of the bladder. The prostate is also enlarged. This tumour had been the occasion of several severe suppressions of urine, and had often been the cause of a failure in drawing off the water with a catheter, by that instrument, most probably, passing into its substance so deep as to hinder the urine entering its openings. The dark line, passing along the tumour from the urethra, was probably made by this means, but now collapsed. A A the cut surfaces of the prostate gland. B B the inner sides of the prostate gland projecting inwards. C the tumour. D the cavity of the bladder.

PLATE XVI.

In this plate is represented the embryo of the chick in the incubated egg, at three different stages of its formation, beginning with the earliest visible appearance of distinct organization. The preparations from which these figures are taken form part of a complete series, contained in Mr. Hunter's collection of comparative anatomy. They are meant to illustrate two positions laid down in this work, viz. That the blood is formed before the vessels, and when coagulated, the vessels appear to arise; that when new vessels are produced in a part, they are not always elongations from the original ones, but vessels newly formed, which afterwards open a communication with the original.

Fig. 1. In this figure the only parts that are distinctly formed are two blood-vessels; on each side of these is a row of small dots or specks of coagulated blood, which are afterwards to become blood-vessels.

Fig. 2. The formation of the embryo is further advanced, vessels appear to be rising up spontaneously in different parts of the membrane; and the specks, out of which they are produced, are in many parts very evident.

Fig. 3. The number of blood-vessels is very considerably increased; they now form a regular system of vessels, composed of larger trunks, and a vast number of ramifications going off from them [a].

a These figures were selected by Mr. Hunter for their present purpose, from an extensive series of drawings of the embryo of the goose at different stages of development, and of which he left only a general account in manuscript, but no detailed descriptions. The above explanations of the figures were doubtless added by the Editor of the original Edition of the ' Treatise on the Blood';—that they are not from the pen of Mr. Hunter, is evident from the fact of there being upwards of ten figures in the original series, showing as many stages of the development of the embryo, *earlier* than that represented in Fig. 1, but with a visible and distinct organization. After a comparison of these figures with the embryo of the fowl and emeu at corresponding stages of development, I would propose the following explanation of them. At the period represented in Fig. 1, red blood is not formed, but although " the heart is beating, it then contains a transparent fluid before any red globules are formed," as Mr. Hunter has justly observed, (vol. iii. p. 66 of the present Edition). The colourless fluid which circulates at this period, when the chick may be compared with the white-blooded invertebrate animals, is not, however, composed entirely, as Mr. Hunter supposed, of the serum and lymph, but contains many colourless globules, smaller than the red-blood-discs of the mature bird, and presenting, under a very high magnifying power, a granular structure like the colourless nuclei of the blood-discs. While, however, the embryo thus exhibits an analogy to the white-blooded animals in the nature of its circulating fluid, it expresses at this, and even at an earlier period, the essential characters of the great division of animals to which it belongs. The row of dots, on each side of the two longitudinal white lines, are the primitive cartilages in which the ossification of

PLATE XVII.

This plate represents a section of the human uterus in the first month after impregnation. The uterus itself is a little enlarged in size, and thickened in its substance; its cavity, everywhere lined with a coagulum of blood, having a smooth internal surface, but adhering firmly to the uterus.

The arteries are injected, to show that it is uncommonly vascular, and vessels are found to be injected in different parts of the coagulum.

The object of this plate is to show the readiness with which vessels are formed in coagulated blood, when attached to a living surface, and its vascularity being to answer useful purposes in the machine; of which this is a remarkable instance, as it is to form the outer membrane of the fœtus, or the connecting medium between it and the uterus.

Fig. 1. A longitudinal section of the uterus, in which the cavity is exposed.

A. The os tincæ projecting into the vagina, of which there is a small portion, to show the length to which the os tincæ projects. B B. The cervix uteri. C C C. The coagulated blood, smooth upon its internal surface, although extremely irregular. D D. The cut surface of the substance of the uterus, which has so intimate a connexion with the coagulum that the one appears to be continued into the other. The laminated appearance is produced by the section of enlarged veins in a collapsed state, which are extremely numerous.

Fig. 2. Is a thin slice of the substance of the uterus and the coagulum adhering to it, dried, and viewed in a microscope, to show the vascularity of the uterus, whose vessels are distinctly seen, continued into the coagulum, and passing about halfway through its substance.

Fig. 3. Is a diagram for the purpose of explaining delusive sensations. (See vol. i. p. 332). A B two portions of the brain. C the seat of the disease, and D the seat of sympathy, which are respectively supplied with the nerves G H, between which passes a communicating nerve F. E the brain.

Fig. 4. Represents an aneurism of the aorta, making its way through the anterior part of the chest. A A the ends of the aorta. B the first sac, which contracted at C, and having proceeded to *d*,

---

the vertebræ commences; and the lines themselves are the folds of the serous layer of the germinal membrane, including the rudiments of the spinal chord and brain; the three divisions of which, viz., medulla oblongata, optic lobes, and cerebral hemispheres, are indicated by the dilatations which succeed each other from behind forwards, towards the anterior or upper end of the embryo. The semicircular white line, surrounding the rudimental head, is the fold of the serous layer of the germinal membrane, forming the circumference of the depression in the yolk, into which the head is beginning to sink. This fold afterwards extends downwards over the dorsal aspect of the embryo, and forms the amnios. The concave edge of the fold thus descending, is slightly indicated near the lower dilated part of the embryo at Fig. 3. The projection on the right side of the embryo (which is seen from behind) opposite the second cerebral enlargement, is the *punctum saliens.* There is little doubt that Mr. Hunter intended this figure to represent the stage at which colourless blood is circulated, as described in the passage above quoted. And it may be observed that this most interesting fact in the history of the development of the vertebrate embryo, has been lately reproduced (by MM. Coste and Delpech), and generally received as a recent discovery.

The 2nd figure illustrates the observation, " The globules do not appear to be formed in those parts of the blood already produced, but rather to rise up in the surrounding parts." The outline of the *punctum saliens,* or rudimental heart, is rendered conspicuous by the red blood which it now circulates : the red globules are aggregated in different parts of the *opake area.* In the third figure the zonular, or terminal sinus is formed, and the circulation of red blood is established in the omphalo-mesenteric vessels, distributed over the yet incomplete vitelline sac. It is obvious from Mr. Hunter's own description, that vessels, and the heart itself, preexist in the embryo to the formation of red globules ; and I have myself observed, in the surrounding opake area, at the period corresponding to that represented in fig. 1., canals already established before the red colouring matter had made its appearance.—R. OWEN.

where it met with resistance from the sternum D D, it became again contracted; but having produced absorption of the sternum *d*, by which an opening was made externally, the sac again expanded. See vol. i. p. 422.

PLATE XVIII.

This represents a front view of the human testicle, upon the body of which is a coagulum of blood adhering to it. For the better understanding this plate it will be necessary to give at length the history of the case.

A man came into St. George's Hospital with an hydrocele, for which he was tapped with a lancet. When the water was evacuated, the testicle was larger to the feel than common, and in a month the tunica vaginalis was as much distended as before the operation. The radical cure was now determined upon; the tunica vaginalis was slit open, but the testicle being enlarged it was thought proper to extract it. Upon the body of the testicle was found a coagulum of blood, resembling a leech in appearance; and in the angle between the testicle and epididymis was another smaller one; at some parts it adhered to the testicle and epididymis, and at others it was loose from both.

The adhesion of the large coagulum was firm, although it admitted of a separation, which was made at one end; when separated, fibres were plainly seen running between it and the testicle. The adhesions of the small coagulum were in many places still firmer. This blood had been extravasated by the puncture made with the lancet in drawing off the water, and had fallen down upon the testicle, where it coagulated.

Over the whole surface of the tunica vaginalis there were vessels filled with blood, and clots of extravasated blood in different parts.

Fig. 1. The testicle, with the tunica vaginalis slit open, exposing its surface.

A A. The body of the testicle. B. A small hydatid arising from its surface, which occurs not unfrequently in that situation, viz. just where the epididymis takes its origin from the testicle. C. The smaller coagulum lying in the angle between the body of the testicle and the epididymis. D. The large coagulum adhering to the body of the testicle. E E E. The tunica vaginalis turned back.

Fig. 2. A portion of the tunica vaginalis magnified to show the appearance of its vessels, and of the small specks of extravasated blood in different parts.

PLATE XIX.

In this plate we have a different view of the same testicle, after the vessels were injected, very much magnified, by which means they were rendered more conspicuous. The whole surface of the testicle now appeared to be a layer of coagulating lymph become vascular.

The surface of adhesion of the larger coagulum was injected for about one twentieth part of an inch, and extremely full of distinct vessels.

The smaller coagulum was in many places injected through and through, in others only for a little way along the surface of adhesion.

A A. The layer of coagulating lymph covering the testicle. B. The hydatid. C C C. The smaller coagulum more exposed than in plate third, and the vessels running upon different parts distinctly seen. The lower portion is detached at one end, and was only vascular at the neck, by which it adhered. D D. The large coagulum. E E E. The tunica vaginalis turned back.

PLATE XX.

Represents two rabbit's ears, one in the natural state, the other in an inflamed state, in consequence of having been frozen and thawed.

The vessels are injected. and as they belonged to the same head, the force applied, and other circumstances, must have been exactly similar.

The difference in the size of the vessels, and the difference in the thickness of the ears themselves, are very evident; but there was an opacity in the inflamed ear compared with the other, which it was not possible to express.

Fig. 1. The ear in its natural state.

A A. The projecting part of the ear.   B. That part which is covered by the skin of the head.
C C C. The principal arterial trunk.

Fig. 2. The inflamed ear.

A A. B. C C C. represent the same parts as in fig. 1.   D. A branch rather larger than the trunk, not distinguishable in the natural state of the ear.

Fig. 3 and 4. Illustrate the growth of bone.   See vol. i. p. 254.

Fig. 5—10. Represent six squares of a glass micrometer, each side of a square being $\frac{1}{300}$ part of an inch.   5, 6, 7, exhibit different appearances of the particles of human blood, their central depression, and the various positions in which they may be seen when rolling down an inclined surface.   8, 9, 10, represent the globules of the blood of a skate, which differ from those of human blood principally in being of a much larger size, in their oval outline, and in the oval figure of their central depression.   See vol. iii. p. 63, note.

PLATE XXI.

Fig. 1. A portion of the ilium taken from the intestines of an ass.   The intestine was in a state of inflammation, and shows the internal surface of the gut partly covered by a layer of coagulating lymph thrown out by the great degree of inflammation which the parts had undergone.

The internal membrane was extremely vascular, and when injected, vessels were seen in portions of the coagulating lymph.   A A. The inner surface of the intestine.   B B. The coagulating lymph which adhered to it.

Fig. 2. The peritoneal coat of a portion of the human intestine, in an inflamed state, to show its vascularity, and to show a small portion of coagulating lymph attached to it by a narrow neck, which is supplied with vessels from it.

Fig. 3—6. Diagrams to explain the action of the valves of the aorta.   See vol. iii. p. 203.

Fig. 3. Shows the artery in its systole, with the three valves nearly close to its sides.   *a a*, a circular section of the aorta.   *b b* the mouths of the coronary arteries, almost covered by, and in the hollow pouch of the valves.   *d* the area within the valves.

Fig. 4. Shows the artery in its diastole, when the three valves run nearly into straight lines, making an equilateral triangle of the area of the aorta.   *a a a* the circular section of the aorta in its state of diastole, being now larger about one fifth.   *b b* the mouths of the coronary arteries, now quite exposed.   *c c c* the hollow pouch of the valves now enlarged.   *d d d* the convexities of the distended valves, filling up the area of artery.   *e c e* the corpora sesamoidea.

Fig. 5. Represents the effect of the heart's systole on the aorta and its valves.   *a a a* a section of the artery in a quiescent state, *b b b* the same in a state of distension.   The valves *a a a* being inextensible retain their original position, while the coats of the artery *b b b* are distended. The former are prevented from assuming a straight line in consequence of the impulsive force of the arterial current, but the effect of their tension in tucking in the sides of the artery is precisely the same.

Fig. 6. Represents the periphery of the aorta the moment the systole of the heart ceases, at which the edges of the valves *a* assume the form of an equilateral triangle.

PLATE XXII.

A ramifying portion of coagulating lymph coughed up from the lungs. The history of the case is as follows :

A man, aged twenty-two, naturally healthy, had his constitution much weakened by a severe course of mercury, which brought on a very violent cough ; he expectorated a quantity of mucus, often mixed with blood. His pulse became so irregular as not to be counted, and he generally felt a cutting pain in his chest.

In a fortnight from this attack, he began coughing up small pieces of coagulating lymph, like worms ; these always produced a fit of coughing in their expulsion, and left an excessive soreness in some part of the chest ; these portions were very numerous, increased in size, and had a branching appearance ; the fits of coughing became also more violent. The specimen here represented was one of the largest ; as they increased in size, the fits became less frequent, and at length disappeared, and the man got well. The patient was under the care of Mr. Saumarez, of Newington Butts, who gave the preparation to Mr. Hunter.

PLATE XXIII.

This represents the uterus and vagina of an ass, on which the experiments were made to produce inflammation upon its internal surface. The inflammation was followed by an exudation of coagulating lymph, an effect which is only produced on the inner surface of a canal opening externally by inflammation in its greatest degree of violence.

The vagina is slit open on the opposite side to that represented in this plate, and the uterus is opened on the exposed side, showing a coagulum, the end of which is in the beginning of the horn ; the other horn is not opened.

A. The vagina slit on the opposite side. B B. The common uterus slit open, which exposes the coagulum. C C. One of the horns of the uterus slit open at its junction with the common cavity, in which lay the extreme end of the coagulum. D. The other horn unopened. E E E E. The coagulum hanging down from the vagina, to which it adhered, but loose at the lower extremity.

PLATE XXIV.

Fig. 1 and 2. "Drawings of two aneurisms: one of the crural artery, (No. 136, *fig.* 1.) which had cured of itself, shown to me by Mr. Ford of Golden Square ; the other of the carotid artery, (No. 136, *fig.* 2.) shown to me by Dr. Baillie."—*Hunterian MS.*

Fig. 1. Represents an aneurism of the right carotid artery, in which the natural process of obliteration, had considerably advanced. *a* the common carotid. *b b* the parietes of the aneurismal sac slit open. *c* a firm old coagulum, completely filling up the cavity of the sac and adhering to it. *d* the internal carotid. *e* the external carotid. The case occurred in 1787, two years after Mr. Hunter's operation, and is described by Dr. Baillie in the *Trans. of a Soc. for the improvement of Med. and Chir. Knowledge,* vol. i. p. 119.

Fig. 2. Represents an aneurism of the right crural artery, the cure of which was completed by the powers of nature. This, Mr. Hunter says, "is the one which had got well, but by what means was not known: or whether it had really been an aneurism or only a contraction of the artery, as I once saw in a young man, a patient in St. George's Hospital, and the small dilatation of the artery took place after the obliteration of the artery, or whether the aneurismal part had contracted to this size, is not now easily ascertained." *a* the cardiac extremity of the crural artery. *b* the contracted sac. *c* the point of contraction. *d* the distal extremity of the crural artery. This case (the case of J. Cathy), described by Mr. Ford in the *Lond. Med. Journal*, vol. ix. p. 144, was seen by Mr. Hunter in September, 1785, three months before he performed his celebrated operation, and is supposed to have been the more immediate cause which suggested it to his mind.

Fig. 3. Representation of an artificial joint with loose cartilages in the cavity. (See vol. iii.) *a* the head of the os humeri. *b* the fractured extremity of the upper portion of the bone. *c* the lower portion of the bone. *d d* the newly formed capsular ligament, surrounding the cavity of the joint. *e e* the surfaces of the fractured ends of the bone, adapted to each other for the purpose of motion ; the upper surface having two concavities with a middle ridge, the lower one being rounded and convex, in some measure fitted to move in either of the cavities. Both these surfaces are partially covered with a substance similar to cartilage, in the interstices of which the bone is exposed.

From the surface of the bones arise a number of small hard projecting parts, very narrow at their base. From the inner surface of the capsular ligament there are excrescences of a softer nature, very large, serrated on their external edge, and attached by narrow necks. Many of these substances, both of the hard and soft kind, were found loose in the cavity, their attachments being broken by the motions of the joint.

Fig. 4. Represents the case of an introsusception. (See vol. iii.) *a* the ilium passing into the introsusception. *b* the portion of the ilium included in the introsusception. *c* the termination of the ilium in the valve of the colon, from which a bougie passes into the intestine. *d* the orifice of the appendix cæci, with a bristle introduced into it. *e e* the course and termination of the appendix cæci. *f f f* the inverted or contained portion of the colon, the inner surface of which has portions of coagulable lymph adhering to it, the consequence of previous inflammation. *g g g* the containing colon laid open, to expose the introsusception. Upon its external surface are the appendiculæ epiploicæ.

PLATE XXV.

Fig. 1. Represents the testes within the abdomen, in an abortive fœtus of about six months. All the intestines, except the rectum, are removed; and the peritonæum in most places is left upon the surfaces which it covers, so that the parts have not that sharpness and distinct appearance which might have been given to them by dissection.

a. The upper part of the object, covered with a cloth. *b b.* The thighs. *c.* The penis. *d.* The scrotum. *e.* The flap of the integuments, abdominal muscles, and peritonæum of the right side, turned back over the os ilium, to bring the testis into view. *f.* The flap of the skin, and cellular membrane of the left side, disposed in the same manner. *g.* The flap of the abdominal muscles, and of the peritonæum of the left side, turned back over the spine of the os ilium. The lower part of this flap is cut away, in order to show the ligament of the testis passing down through the ring into the scrotum. *h h.* The lower part of each kidney. *i.* The projection formed by the lower vertebræ lumborum, and by the bifurcation of the aorta and vena cava. *k.* The rectum filled with meconium, and tied at its upper part, where the colon was cut away. *l.* That branch of the inferior mesenteric artery which was going to the colon. *m.* The lower branch of the same artery, which went down into the pelvis, behind the rectum. *n.* The posterior surface of the cavity of the bladder; the anterior part, which is higher than the ossa pubis in so young a fœtus, being cut away. *o o.* The hypogastric, or umbilical, arteries cut through, where they were turning up by the sides of the bladder, in their way to the navel. *p. p.* The ureter of each side passing down before the psoas muscle and iliac vessels, in its course to the lower part of the bladder. *q q.* The spermatic arteries running a little serpentine. *r r.* The testes situated before the psoæ muscles, a little higher than the inguina. In this figure the interior edge of the testis is turned a little outwards, to show the spermatic vessels coming forwards to the posterior edge of the testis, in the duplicature of the peritonæum, which duplicature connects the testis, incloses its vessels, and gives it an external smooth coat, much after the same manner as the duplicature of the mesentery connects the intestine, conveys its vessels, and gives it a polished covering.

The beginning of the epididymis is seen at the upper end of the testis, from which it runs down on the outside (and therefore in this view behind the body) of the testis.

s s. The vas deferens of each side, passing across, in a serpentine course, from the extremity of the epididymis, at the outside of the lower end of the testis, and then before the lower part of the ureter, in its way to the vesicula seminalis. *t t.* What I have called the gubernacula or ligaments of the testis in a fœtus. On the left side this ligament is entire, and exposed in its whole length, the rings, skin of the groin and scrotum being removed, so that it is seen going down from the lower end of the testis into the scrotum; but on the right side its upper and fore part is cut away, that the continuity of the epididymis and vas deferens may be seen; and no more of the ligament is exhibited than what is situated within the cavity of the abdomen.

N. B. The lower part of the ligament, as it is seen in the right side of this figure, lies so loose in the passage through the muscles, and is there so loosely covered by the peritonæum, that when the testis is pulled up, more of the ligament is seen within the cavity of the abdomen, and then the peritonæum is made tight and smooth at that place; but on the contrary, when the scrotum is pulled downwards, the lower part of the ligament is dragged some way down through the passage in the muscles, and the loose peritonæum is carried along with it; so that then there is a small elongation of that membrane, with an orifice from the cavity of the belly like the mouth of a small hernial sac, on the fore part of the ligament.

Fig. 2. represents the testes, &c., in the same subject as Plate XXVI.; all the parts above the ossa ilium being removed, and the abdominal muscles of the left side turned down to show the opening of the sac into, or from the abdomen; the bladder being likewise turned downwards to show the vasa deferentia winding round behind it.

a a. The thighs unfinished. *b.* The penis. *c.* The middle part of the scrotum; its lateral parts being removed, to show the testes. *d d.* The skin and cellular membrane of the abdomen turned down over the thighs. *e e.* Part of the abdominal muscles and peritonæum turned down at each groin. *f f.* The peritonæum covering the iliacus internus muscle of each side. *g.* The intestinum rectum filled with meconium. *h.* The bladder with the umbilical artery on each side of it, turned a little forwards over the symphysis of the pubis. *i i.* The ureters passing over the iliac vessels to the pelvis. *k.* The right testis exposed, as in Fig. 2. *v. w. x x. y.* *l.* The left testis in the inclosed process of the peritonæum. See Fig. 2. *u.* *m.* The spermatic vessels of the left side, seen through the peritonæum which covers them, in their descent through the abdominal muscles at the groin. *n.* The left vas deferens seen through the peritonæum, in its passage from the mouth of the sac to the posterior part of the bladder. *o.* The mouth, or aperture of the process of the peritonæum, whereby its mouth or cavity communicates with the general cavity of the belly. This aperture closes up, and the membrane becomes smooth at this place, when the fœtus grows a little older; unless when the gut falls down after the testis, and keeps it open; in that case it makes the mouth of the hernial sac. *p*. The left epigastric artery branching upon the inside of the rectus muscle, which is here turned downwards and outwards. This artery is always situated, as in this figure, on the inside of the mouth of the hernial sac, or passage of the spermatic vessels.

N.B. It is evident that part of the peritonæum, which in this figure is carried down in the form of a hernial sac to a little below the testis, lies before the testis, epididymis, spermatic vessels, and vas deferens; and that it covers those parts in the same manner as it covers the abdominal viscera, viz., the posterior part of the sac (supposing the sac to be cut lengthways into two halves,) is united with them, and gives them a smooth surface; while the anterior half of the sac lies loose before them, and may be removed to some distance from them, as when the sac is distended with water.

PLATE XXVI.

This figure represents nearly the same parts in a fœtus somewhat older than Fig. 1. Plate XXV., in order to show the state of the testes when they have recently descended from the abdomen into the scrotum. The small intestines are removed, and the large intestines are left in their natural situation, not now obstructing the view of the testes. On the left side the integuments only are removed, which shows the chord passing out through the ring, with the testicle in the vaginal coat. On the right the ring is cut through, and the whole vaginal coat is slit open, exposing the testicle and chord.

a a. The liver in outlines. *b b*. The thighs unfinished. *c*. The penis. *d*. The middle part of the scrotum; on each side of which the fore part of the scrotum is cut away, that the testes may be seen. *e e*. The two flaps of the skin, and of the cellular membrane, dissected off from the lower part of the abdomen, and turned down upon the thighs. *f*. The intestinum cæcum. *g g*. The appendicula cæci vermiformis. *h*. The arch of the colon. *i*. The turn of the colon under the spleen. *k*. The colon passing down on the outside of the left kidney. *l*. The last turn of the colon, commonly called its sigmoid flexure, which in adults is seated quite in the cavity of the pelvis. *m*. The beginning of the rectum. *n*. Part of the abdominal muscles of the right side, with the smooth investing peritonæum, turned out over the spine of the os ilium. *o o*. The lower part of the obliquus externus muscle of the left side. *p*. The lower part of the rectus muscle of the right side, turned outwards and towards the left side, so that the epigastric artery is seen going to the inside of that muscle. *q*. The fore part of the bladder. *r*. The urachus (as it is called). *s*. The crural vessels coming into the thigh from behind the ligamentum Fallopii. *t*. The external appearance of the spermatic rope of the left side. *u*. The external appearance of the testis, when its tunica vaginalis, or process of the peritonæum, is a little distended with air or water, poured into it from the cavity of the abdomen. *v*. The right testis, brought fully into view by laying open the process of the peritonæum in its whole length. *w*. The head of the epididymis, of the same side. *x x*. The spermatic vessels. *y*. The vas deferens. *z*. The ureter. &. The remains of the gubernaculum, or ligament, which bound and conducted the testis to the scrotum.

PLATE XXVI*.

A side view of the pelvis of a young ram, to show the right testicle remaining in the cavity of the abdomen, after the left had come down, but which is removed with that half of the pelvis.

The testicle which lies in the loins is flatter than common, and is only attached by one edge, which is principally by the epididymis; there is also a ligament passing from the upper part of the common attachment which binds the testicle to the posterior part of the abdominal muscles; this is analogous to the ligament that attaches the ovarium to the same part in the female quadruped.

The epididymis passes along the outer or posterior edge; and at the lower part becomes larger and pendulous, making a little twist upon itself where it becomes vas deferens.

The vas deferens is a little contorted, and passes down obliquely over the psoas muscle to the bladder.

From the lower end of the testicle there is a ridge continued along the psoas muscle through the abdominal ring, going on to the scrotum, which is most probably the gubernaculum; but it was so much covered by a hard suety fat, that I could not exactly ascertain its structure: at the lower part of this ridge, about an inch and a half from the ring, I found the termination of the cremaster, which was a tolerably large muscle; part of its fibres seemed to arise in common with the internal oblique, while the rest appeared to come from the psoas and iliacus internus behind it; the outer portion passed inwards and downwards, and spread upon the forepart of the ridge, or gubernaculum, where the greatest part of its fibres were lost, and the rest of them were continued into the back part of it. The posterior portion got upon the inside of the ridge and was lost in the same manner as the former. A the inside of the thigh, only having the outline drawn. B B the inside of the abdominal muscles spread out. C the symphysis of the os pubis. D the muscles of the thigh cut through at their origin where they arise from a middle tendon. E the lower end of the right kidney. F G the iliac vessels exposed to show their situation. H the remains of the umbilical artery. I the urinary bladder. K the body of the right testicle, with the ramifications of the veins upon the surface. L the epididymis. M the vas deferens. N the vesiculæ, commonly called seminales.

PLATE XXVII.

Shows two testicles, with the spermatic chords dissected; in the one the vas deferens, in the other a portion of the epididymis, is wanting.

Fig. 1. The right testicle and spermatic chord.

A A. The body of the testicle. B B. The spermatic chord, in which there is no appearance of vas deferens. C. The epididymis, where it takes its origin from the body of the testicle. D. The abrupt termination of the epididymis, it not being continued to the lower end of the testicle.

Fig. 2. The left testicle.

A A. The body of the testicle. B. The blood-vessels of the testicle separated from the vas deferens. C. The origin of the epididymis. D. The termination of the epididymis; to show which, the tunica vaginalis is removed. E. The origin of the vas deferens. F. The vas deferens, as it passes up towards the ring of the abdominal muscles.

PLATE XXVIII.

A side view of the pelvis, taken from the same subject as Plate XXVII., in which the vasa deferentia did not communicate with the vesiculæ, and the vesiculæ, did not communicate with the urethra. A the body of the penis. B the symphysis of the pubis. C the bladder. D the left ureter. E E the rectum. F the anus. G the sphincter muscle of the anus, turned aside. H the levator muscle of the anus, turned down. I the prostate gland. K the Cowper's gland of the left side. L the peritoneum, which lined the left side of the pelvis. M the sacrum, where it is articulated with the os ilium. N the left vas deferens. O the vesiculæ.

PLATE XXIX.

To show the gradual increase, in size, of the testes of the sparrow, from the middle of winter to the beginning of the breeding season, I examined those glands in January, February, March and April; and the appearances they put on at these different periods are faithfully represented in the Plate, with the date of their examination annexed to each.

If we compare their size in January, with what it is in April, it hardly appears possible that such a wonderful change could have taken place during so short a period.

PLATE XXX.

This Plate is a representation of Mr. Wright's free martin, taken from a drawing of the living animal, by Mr. Gilpin. It shows the external form of that animal, which is neither like the bull nor cow; but resembling the ox or spayed heifer.

PLATE XXXI.

This Plate represents the organs of generation of Mr. Wright's free martin, which are more the parts of a bull than those of a cow; and the animal, while alive, had a good deal the character and look of an ox. A the peak of the labia. B B the labia. C the glans clitoridis. D D D D the inner surface of the common vagina. E E the orifices of the ducts of two glands. (The glandular sinuses of Malpighi and Gaertner.) F meatus urinarius. G G the inner surface of the true vagina, terminating in a blind end at H. H the termination of the vagina in a blind end. I I I I what may be called uterus, but impervious. K K what may be called horns of the uterus. L L the testicles. M M the spermatic vessels. N N the cremaster muscles. O O the vesiculæ seminales. P P the ducts of the vesiculæ seminales seen through the vagina. Q points to the ducts of ditto, into which are introduced bristles[a].

PLATE XXXII.

This plate shows the organs of generation of Mr. Arbuthnot's free martin, which are almost a complete mixture of the male and female: with this structure of the parts, the external appearances and general character of the animal corresponded, it being neither that of the bull nor cow, but a mixt character. A the peak of the labia. B B the two labia. C the glans clitoridis. D D the inside of the common vagina. E E orifices of the ducts of two glands. (The glandular canals of Malpighi and Gaertner.) F the orifice of the meatus urinarius. G G the true vagina. H H either the contracted vagina, or what may be called uterus. I I the horns of ditto, only pervious a little way. K the right ovarium deprived of its capsula. L the left ovarium inclosed in its capsula. M a bristle introduced through the orifice into the capsula. N the right testicle. O O O O the right vas deferens. P P the vesiculæ seminales. Q Q the ducts of vesiculæ seminales seen through the vagina. R points to the openings of the vasa deferentia and vesiculæ seminales.

---

[a] This description, it will be seen in the 2nd edition of the Animal Economy, is made to apply to Plate XXXII., and *vice versâ*, in consequence of an alteration in the relative position of the plates in that edition which was unaccompanied with a corresponding change in the letter-press. The error resulting from this oversight is corrected in the present edition.

PLATE XXXIII.

This plate exhibits a front view of the organs of generation of Mr. Well's free martin, which are more the parts of a cow than of a bull; and the animal itself resembled a young heifer very much in its appearance. A the clitoris. B B the crura clitoridis. C the urethra. D the bladder. E the body of the uterus beyond the bladder, which is impervious. F F the horns of ditto, which are also impervious. G the left ovarium deprived of its capsula. H the capsula inclosing its ovarium. I I I I interrupted parts of the vasa deferentia. K K the spermatic vessels. L the gubernaculum of the right side. M the beginning of the tunica vaginalis communis, into which is introduced a bristle to show that it is hollow. N N Vessels going behind the bladder. O O the two ureters. P P the vesiculæ seminales.

PLATE XXXIV.

Fig. 1. A part of a uterus at the ninth month of utero-gestation, with a portion of the placenta, to show the mode in which the blood-vessels of the mother communicate with it.

A. The substance of the uterus, separated from the placenta, and turned back. B. The surface of the placenta by which it is attached to the uterus, covered by the decidua. C. The angle of reflection, at which the uterus is turned back upon itself. E. The edge of the placenta. E. The decidua covering the chorion.

Upon the surface of the uterus are to be seen the veins or sinuses, running in an oblique direction, filled with wax, and broken off where they pass through the decidua.

a a a a. The arteries injected and broken off as they pass from the uterus to the placenta. *b b b b.* The continuation of these arteries, which make several spiral turns as they dip into the decidua, and afterwards terminate on the surface of the placenta. *c c c c.* The veins injected and broken off where they pass into the substance of the uterus. *d d d d.* The corresponding portions of the same veins, where they pass from the placenta through the decidua. *e e e e.* The blood-vessels, ramifying upon the decidua, broken off from the uterus.

Fig. 2. Is a section of the placenta of the monkey figured in Plates XXXV. and XXXVI.

a. The cut surface, showing the fissure passing into the substance of the placenta from the uterine surface. *b.* The surface which adhered to the uterus, on which is the open end of a vein broken off, which was passing from the placenta to the uterus. *c c.* The cut ends of the vessels of the umbilical chord as they were ramifying on the inner surface of the placenta.

PLATE XXXV.

The bilobed placenta of a monkey, showing the fœtal surface with the membranes attached and extended beyond its circumference. The fœtal vessels ramify over the surface as in the human subject, and the chord is attached near to the edge of the placenta, as it often is in the human subject, but it is more regularly twisted. The amnios, which covers as usual the fœtal surface of the placenta, is thrown into wrinkles near the chord and where it passes over the interlobular fissures.

PLATE XXXVI.

The same placenta, showing the uterine surface, with part of the decidua and other membranes attached to it.

a. The decidua reflected from the chorion and placenta. *b.* The chorion, which is attached to the outer surface of the placenta. *c.* The amnios. *dddd.* The broken ends of the veins, which return the blood from the cells of the maternal placenta to the uterine sinuses. (See fig. 2. pl. XXXIV. which is a section of the same placenta.)

PLATE XXXVII.

A portion of intestine of a hog, the peritoneal coat of which is covered in several places with small pellucid cysts containing air.

It was sent to me by my friend Mr. Jenner, surgeon, at Berkley, who informed me, that this appearance is found very frequently upon the intestines of hogs that are killed in the summer months. A. The portion of the mesentery. B. The portion of intestine on which the air-cells are situated.

PLATE XXXVIII.

The crop, taken from a pigeon when it had no young ones. The crop in the pigeon is probably more in the middle of the neck than in any other bird, being two equal bags, as it were, passing out, laterally, from the œsophagus; while in most other birds it is a little on one side. The œsophagus of those birds who have crops, may be divided into two, a superior and inferior. The superior is that which leads from the mouth to the crop; the inferior, from the crop to the gizzard.

The crop was inverted and distended with spirits. It shows the appearance of its internal surface

A. The inner surface of the superior œsophagus. B B. The inside of the two projecting bags of the crop. C. The inferior œsophagus, leading from the crop to the gizzard. D D D D. Glands situated on the lower part of the crop, and continued into the inferior œsophagus. E. A glandular structure upon the inner surface of this œsophagus, just before it terminates in the gizzard, for the purpose of secreting a substance analogous to the gastric liquor.

PLATE XXXIX.

The crop from a male pigeon, while the female was breeding, to show the change which takes place at that time, on its internal surface, for the purpose of secreting a substance which is to nourish the young.

The crop is prepared in the same way as in Plate XXXVIII.; and the only difference in the appearance is the glandular structure on the inner surface of the two lateral projecting bags, which is not seen at any other time.

PLATE XL.

A thermometer which has the scale so constructed as to admit of its being introduced into any cavity that can receive the ball. The scale is moveable; but the freezing point is marked on the stem or glass.

Fig. 1. A front view, exposing the glass stem of the thermometer, through which the divisions marked upon the concave surface of the sliding ivory scale which embraces it, are very distinctly seen.

a. The freezing point, which is marked upon the stem by a scratch on the glass.

Fig. 2. A side view, showing the degrees marked near the edge of the convex side of the ivory scale.

The thermometer is to be adjusted for measuring high or low degrees of heat, by bringing any number marked upon the scale opposite the freezing point, and counting either upwards or downwards.

PLATE XLI.

The olfactory, or first pair of nerves, as they are seen upon the membrane of the septum narium.

The bony septum is removed to expose the nerves of the right nostril, as they pass at first between the membrane and bone. A. the os frontis. B. the frontal sinus. C. the cartilaginous part of the septum narium. **** the cut edge, from which the septum has been separated all round. D. the surface of the common skin, where it is lost in the membrane of the nose. E. the upper lip. F. part of the alveolar process of the maxillary bone next the symphysis. G. the roof of the mouth. H. the bony palate. I. the uvula and palatum molle. K. the upper part of the fauces. L. the opening of the Eustachian tube. M. the cuneiform process of the os occipitis. N. the inside of the cuneiform process, near the foramen magnum occipitale. O. The posterior clinoid process. P. The sphenoid sinus, with its septum. Q. The cella Turcica. R. The crista galli. S S. The membrane of the right nostril that lined the septum; the septum being removed. T. A branch of the fifth pair of nerves, that comes through the foramen commune or spheno-palatinum. U U U. The first pair of nerves, having passed through the cribriform plate of the ethmoid bone, ramifying on the membrane of the septum.

PLATE XLII.

The olfactory, or first pair of nerves, as they are seen upon the membrane of the nose, which covers the turbinated bones; the exterior parts of the face being removed.

This engraving was taken from the same head as plate XLI. A. The os frontis. B. The os nasi. C. The cartilaginous and membranous part of the nose. D. The ala nasi, with the skin left on. E. The septum narium. F. The upper lip. G. The cut surface. H H H. The alveolar process of the superior maxillary bone. I. Part of the antrum. K. The os occipitis. L. The body of the sphenoid bone. M. The groove made by the carotid artery. N. The posterior clinoid process. O. the sphenoid sinus. P. The crista galli. Q. The membrane of the nose. R. The membrane, a little more convex, where the inferior turbinated bone is situated. S. The same where the superior turbinated bone is situated. T. The branch of the fifth pair of nerves that was supposed to be lost on the membrane of the nose. U U U. The trunk of the first pair of nerves which is afterwards lost upon that part of Schneider's membrane that covers the turbinated bones.

PLATE XLIII.

Fig. 1. A transverse section of the crystalline humour of the eye of a cuttle-fish, to show its structure; the central part is transparent, but the others are opaque, having been coagulated by proof spirits; and for the appearance of distinct fibres surrounding the central part.

These fibres are not uniform circles or ovals, since the layers are of different thicknesses in particular parts. *a a.* The fibres where they are most numerous. *b b.* Where they are least so.

Fig. 2. A section of the crystalline humour, the central part being removed, to show the fibrous structure of the surrounding laminæ.

PLATE XLIV.

This fish is called a Grampus [a]; it was caught at the mouth of the river Thames, in the year 1759, and brought up to Westminster Bridge in a barge. It was twenty-four feet long.

---

[a] [*Phocœna Orca,* Cuv. *Delphinus Orca,* Linn. This is acknowledged to be the most accurate figure of the Grampus hitherto published; and is cited by M. Fred. Cuvier as the type of that species. See *Histoire de sCétacés,* 8vo. 1836, p. 177.]

PLATE XLV.

Another species of Grampus [a], which was caught in the river Thames, fifteen years ago. It was eighteen feet long.

PLATE XLVI.

Fig. 1. A species of Bottle-nosed Whale; the *Delphinus Delphis* of Linnæus [b]. It was caught upon the sea-coast, near Berkeley, where it had been seen for several days, following its mother, and was taken along with the old one, and sent up to me whole, for examination, by Mr. Jenner, Surgeon, at Berkeley. The old one was eleven feet long.

Fig. 2. The head of the same Whale as fig. 1. to show the shape of the blow-hole, which is transverse, and almost semicircular.

PLATE XLVII.

The Bottle-nose [d] Whale described by Dale [c]. It is similar to that of Plate XLVI. in its general form, but has only two small pointed teeth in the fore part of the upper jaw, and is rather lighter coloured on the belly. It was caught above London Bridge in the year 1783, and became the property of the late Mr. Alderman Pugh, who very politely allowed me to examine its structure, and to take away the bones. It was twenty-one feet long.

PLATE XLVIII.

Fig. 1. The *Balæna rostrata* of FABRICIUS, or Piked Whale [d]. It was caught upon the Dogger Bank. It had met with some accident between the lower jaws under the tongue, in which part a considerable collection of air had taken place, so as to raise up the tongue and its attachments into a round body in the mouth, projecting even beyond the jaws. This rendered the head specifically lighter than the water, so that it could not sink, and therefore was easily caught. It was seventeen feet long, and was brought to St. George's Fields, where I purchased it. The dorsal fin having been cut off close to the back, is therefore only marked by a dotted line.

Fig. 2. A view of the tail, to show its breadth.

PLATE XLIX.

Includes the external parts of generation, with the relative situation of the anus and the nipples, of the *Balæna rostrata.*

I have searched in vain among the existing documents, relating to Mr. Hunter's researches on the Cetacea, for any note or memorandum tending to authenticate the above description. The original drawing, coloured after nature, exists in the Hunterian Collection, and is marked 'Porpus'. It is unnecessary to observe to those who have examined the common Porpoise, (*Phocæna communis,* Cuv.) that the figure in Plate XLV. is an exact representation of that species.

[b] [This is the *Delphinus Tursio* of Fabricius, the '*Grand Dauphin*' or *Souffleur* of Cuvier; and a larger species than the *Delph. Delphis,* Linn., but with fewer teeth, having from 21 to 23 obtuse conical teeth on each side of each jaw, while the *Delph. Delphis* has double that number.]

[c] [*Delphinus Dalei,* Cuv. *Delphinus bidens,* Schreber. *Hyperoodon Dalei,* Lacépede. *Heterodon Hunteri,* Lesson. See De Blainville, "Note sur un Cétacé échoué au Havre," in the Bulletin de la Société Philomathique, September 1835, which relates to the same species.]

[d] [The young of the great Northern Rorqual, (*Balæna Boops,* Linn.) according to Cuvier; but regarded as a smaller and distinct species by Lacépede and other naturalists, and called *Balænoptera rostrata.*]

Fig. 1. The labia pudendi spread open, exposing the meatus urinarius, vagina, and anus, which in a natural state are all concealed, there only appearing a long slit, the two edges of which are in contact.

A A. The labia pudendi. B. The clitoris. C. The meatus urinarius. D. The opening of the vagina. E. The anus.

Fig. 2. The sulcus, in which the left nipple lies, spread open, and the nipple itself exposed to view.

Fig. 3. The sulcus of the right nipple, in a natural state, only appearing like a line.

Fig. 4. A sulcus near to the nipple, which is spread open to show the inside. This sulcus, I conceive, gives a freedom to the motion of the skin of these parts, so as to allow the nipple to be more freely exposed.

Fig. 5. The same sulcus on the opposite side, closed up.

PLATE L.

A side view of one of the plates of whalebone of the *Balæna rostrata*. A. The part of the plate which projects beyond the gum. B. The portion which is sunk into the gum. C C. A white substance, which surrounds the whalebone, forming there a projecting bead, and also passing between the plates, to form their external lamellæ. D D. The part analogous to the gum. E. A fleshy substance, covering the jaw bone, and on which the inner lamella of the plate is formed. F. The termination of the plate of whalebone in a kind of hair.

PLATE LI.

Fig. 1. A perpendicular section of several plates of whalebone in their natural situation in the gum : their inner edges, or shortest terminations, are removed, and the cut edges of the plates seen from the inside of the mouth. The upper part shows the rough surface formed by the hairy termination of each plate of whalebone. The middle part shows the distance the plates of whalebone are from each other. The lower part shows the white substance in which they grow, and also the basis on which they stand.

Fig. 2. An outline considerably magnified, to show the mode of growth of the plates, and of the white intermediate substance.

A. The middle layer of the plate, which is formed upon a pulp or cone that passes up in the centre of the plate. The termination of this layer forms the hair. B. One of the outer layers, which grows, or is formed, from the intermediate white substance. C C C C. The intermediate white substance, laminæ of which are continued along the middle layer, and form the substance of the plate of whalebone. D. The outline of another plate of whalebone. E. The basis on which the plates are formed, which adheres to the jaw bone.

PLATE LII.

Two specimens of Siren, or Mud Iguana from South Carolina[a].

" The lesser one B, which is preserved in spirits, measures about nine inches in length, and appears to be a very young state of the animal, as we may observe from the fin of the tail, and the opercula or coverings of the gills being not yet extended to their full size. These opercula, in their present state, consist each of three indented lobes hiding the gills from view, and are placed just above the

[a] [*Siren lacertina*, Linn., Cuv.]

two feet. These feet appear like little arms and hands, each furnished with four fingers, and each finger with a claw.

In the specimen A, which is thirty-one inches long, the head is something like an eel, but more compressed; the eyes are small, and placed as those of the eel are; in this they are scarce visible. This smallness of the eye best suits an animal that lives so much in the mud. The nostrils are very plainly to be distinguished; these, with the gills, and the remarkable length of the lungs, show it to be a true amphibious animal. The mouth is small in proportion to the body; but its palate and inside of the lower jaw (see Fig. C), are well provided with many rows of pointed teeth; with this provision of nature, added to the sharp exterior bony edges of both the upper and under jaw, the animal seems capable of biting and grinding the hardest kind of food. The skin, which is black, is full of small scales resembling chagrin. These scales are of different sizes and shapes according to their situation, but all appear sunk into its gelatinous surface: those along the back and belly are of an oblong oval form, and close set together: in the other parts they are round, and more distinct. Both the sides are mottled with small white spots, and have two distinct lines composed of small white streaks, continued along from the feet to the tail. The fin of the tail has no rays, and is no more than an adipose membrane like that of the eel; this fin appears more distinctly in the dry animal than in those that have been preserved in spirits.

The opercula or coverings to the gills in dry specimens appear shrivelled up, but yet we may plainly see that they have been doubly pennated. Under these coverings are the openings to the gills, three on each side, agreeable to the number of the opercula. In the plate at Fig. F the fins are represented as they appear when just taken out of the water and put into spirits of wine.

The form of these pennated coverings approach very nearly to what I have some time ago observed in the larva or aquatic state of our English Lacerta, known by the name of Eft or Newt (see Fig. D and E), which serve them for coverings to their gills, and for fins to swim with during this state; and which they lose, as well as the fin of their tails, when they change their state and become land animals; as I have observed by keeping them alive for some time myself."—*From Mr. Ellis's paper in the Phil. Trans., Vol. LVI., p.* 189.

PLATE LIII.

Male and Female TORPEDO [a]

Fig. 1. A view of the under surface of the female.

a. An exposure, on flaying off the skin, of the right electric organ, which consists of white pliant columns, in a close and for the most part hexagonal arrangement, giving the general appearance of a honey-comb in miniature. These columns have been sometimes denominated cylinders; but, having no interstices, they are all angular, and chiefly six-cornered. *b.* The skin which covered the organ, showing on its inward side an hexagonal net work. *c.* The nostrils in the form of a crescent. *d.* The mouth in a crescent contrary to that of the nostrils, furnished with several rows of very small hooked teeth. *e.* The bronchial apertures, five on each side. *f.* The place of the heart. *g g g.* The place of the two anterior transverse cartilages, which, passing one above and the other below the spine, support the diaphragm, and uniting towards their extremities, form on either side a kind of clavicle and scapula. *h h.* The outward margin of the great lateral fin. *i i.* Its inner margin, confining with the electric organ. *k.* The articulation of the great lateral fin with the scapula. *l.* The abdomen. *m m m.* The place of the posterior transverse cartilage which is single, united with the spine, and supports on each side the smaller lateral fins. *n n n n.* The two smaller lateral fins. *o.* The anus. *p.* The fin of the tail.

[a] *Torpedo Narke,* Cuv.

Fig. 2. A view of the upper surface of the female.

a a. An exposure of the upper part of the right electric organ. *b.* The skin which covered the organ. *c.* The eyes, prominent and looking horizontally outwards, but capable of being occasionally withdrawn into their sockets. *d.* Two circular apertures communicating with the mouth, and furnished each with a membrane, which in air, as well as in water, plays regularly backwards and forwards across the aperture in the office of inspiration. *e.* The place of the right branchiæ. *f.* The two fins of the back. *g g.* The place of the anterior transverse cartilages.

Fig. 3. A view of the under surface of the male, whose size, as here represented, is, in general, smaller than that of the female.

a a. Two appendices, distinguishing the male species.

PLATE LIV.

Electric Organs of the Torpedo.

Fig. 1. The upper surface of the electric organ.

A A. The common skin of the animal. B. The inspiratory opening. C. The eye. D. The part in which the gills are inclosed. E E E. The skin dissected off from the electric organ, and turned outwards; the honey-comb appearance on its internal surface corresponding with the upper surface of the organ. F. The part of the skin which covered the gills, with some ramifications of an excretory duct upon it. G G G. The upper surface of the electric organ, formed by the upper extremities of the perpendicular columns.

Fig. 2. The right electric organ divided horizontally into nearly two equal parts at the place where the nerves enter; the upper half being turned outwards.

A A. B B. C C. D D. The corresponding parts of the trunks of the nerves, as they emerge from the gills, and ramify in the electric organ. A A. The first or anterior trunk arising just before the gills. B B. The second or middle trunk arising behind the first gill. C C. The anterior branch of the third trunk arising behind the second gill. D D. The posterior branch of the third trunk arising behind the third gill.

Fig. 3. A perpendicular section of the Torpedo a little below its inspiratory openings.

A A. The upper surface of the fish. B B. The muscles of the back as divided by the section. C. The medulla spinalis. D. The œsophagus. E. The left gill split, to expose the course of a trunk of the nerve through it. F. The breathing surface of the right gill. G G. The fins. H H. The perpendicular columns which compose the electric organ, with a representation of their horizontal partitions. I. One of the trunks of the nerves, with its ramifications.

PLATE LV.

Gymnotus Electricus.

Fig. 1. Shows the whole animal of the full size. It lies on one side; which posture exposes the whole of the under fin. The head is twisted, to show its upper part, on which are seen the eyes, &c.

Fig. 2. Shows the animal lying in the same position; but the head is twisted in the contrary direction, so as to expose its under surface. Between the two fins, and before the beginning of the under fin, is the cavity of the belly of the fish; at the anterior part of which cavity is the anus.

PLATE LVI.

Electric Organs, GYMNOTUS.

Fig. 3. This figure exhibits the whole of the two organs on one side, the skin being removed as far as these organs extend.

A. The lower surface of the head of the animal. B. The cavity of the belly. C. The anus. D. The pectoral fin. E. The back of the fish where the skin has not been removed. F F. The fin which runs along the lower edge of the fish. G G G. The skin turned back. H H H. The lateral muscles of the above fin removed and carried back with the skin, to expose the small organ. I. Part of the muscle left in its place. K K K. The large organ. L L L. The small organ. M M M. The substance which divides the large organ from the small. N. At this place the above substance is removed.

PLATE LVII.

Fig. 4. A section of the whole thickness of the fish near the upper part, a little magnified. The skin is removed as far back as the posterior edge of the organ, and the other parts immediately belonging to it, such as the medulla spinalis. There are several pieces or sections taken out of the organ, which expose everything that has any relation to it. At the two ends of the figure, F F, the organ is entire, the skin only being removed. A A. The body of the animal near the back, covered by the skin. B B. The belly-fin, covered also by the skin. C. Part of the skin removed from the organ and turned back. D D. The muscles which move the fin laterally, and which immediately cover the small organ. E. The middle muscles of the fin, which lie immediately between the two small organs. F F. The outer surface of the large organ, as it appears when the skin is removed. G. The small organ, as it appears when the lateral muscles are removed. H H. The cut ends of the muscles of the back, which have been removed to expose the deeper seated parts. I I. The cut ends of the large organ, part of which has also been removed to expose the deeper seated parts. K. The cut end of the small organ. L. A part of the large organ, the rest having been removed. M. The cut end of the above part. N. A section of the small organ. O O. The middle partition which divides the two large organs. P. A fatty membrane, which divides the large organ from the small. Q. The air-bladder. R. The nerves going to the organ. S. The medulla spinalis. T. The singular nerve (*nervus lateralis*).

Fig. 5. A transverse section of the fish, exposing at one view all the parts of which it is composed.

A. The external surface of the side of the fish. B. The under fin. C C C C. The cut ends of the muscles of the back. D. The cavity of the air-bladder. E. The body of the spine. F. The medulla spinalis. G. The large artery and vein. H H. The cut ends of the two large organs. I I. The cut ends of the two small organs. K. The partition between the organs.

PLATE LVIII.

ANIMAL FLOWER OF BARBADOES (*Serpula gigantea*, Pallas).

Fig. 1. A drawing of the animal after death, as it appeared in spirits, a little magnified.

A. The under side of the body. B B. The cartilages which attach the animal to the sides of the cavity in which it lies. C. One of the cones covered by its membrane, in a collapsed state. D. The lowest spiral turn of the membrane, and its tentacula spread out. E E. The cut edges of the divided membrane, which are turned on each side to show the cone. F. The cone as it appears in the intervals between the spiral turns of the membrane. G. The moveable shell, with the smooth cartilaginous covering in an outside view. H. The flattened end of the moveable shell, with hair upon it. I I. The two claws that arise from the surface of the flattened end of the moveable shell. K. The anus, into which a hog's bristle is inserted.

Fig. 2. A drawing of the animal, with its tentacula expanded in search of food, as it appears in the sea; taken from a sketch made in Barbadoes, where no draughtsman could be procured while the animal was alive. This also is larger than the animal.

a. The sort of brainstone in which the animal was discovered. *b.* The external prominent shell. *c c.* The membrane which is protruded with the cones and immoveable shell, and makes a fold over the edges of the prominent shell. *d d.* The membranes and tentacula in a state of expansion. *e.* The inner side of the moveable shell, as it appears when protruded. *f.* The hole in the brainstone, as it appears when the prominent shell is broken off, and which may be seen in many specimens of brainstone.

PLATE LIX.

Fig. 1. One of the incrusted skulls sent over by the Margrave of Anspach, which is much larger than that of the common white bear, longer for its breadth, and having a greater hollow between the anterior part of the skull and the bones of the face[a].

Fig. 2. Another skull, which differs in many respects from fig. 1, and nearly in the same degree that the first does from the skull of the recent white bear[b].

PLATE LX.

Fig. 1. A portion of a skull; to what animal it belongs is not exactly ascertained, unless it be the growing state of the bones in one of the varieties of the white bear species, but it is materially different from the full-grown skulls expressed in Plate LIX. It is rather too large in proportion to the others[c].

Fig. 2. Two of the incrusted ossa humeri, to show that these bones vary very much among themselves, these two being in many respects dissimilar[d].

[a] This belongs to the extinct species called *Ursus spelæus* by Cuvier.

[b] This is the *Ursus arctoideus* of Cuvier.

[c] This fragment appears to belong to the extinct bear called *Ursus priscus* by Goldfuss.

[d] One of the most marked differences is that the internal condyle is perforated in one of the humeri (though not represented in the plate), showing an analogy to the cat tribe, while in the other it is imperforate as in the existing bears.

THE END.

PRINTED BY RICHARD AND JOHN E. TAYLOR,
RED LION COURT, FLEET STREET.

PLATE I.

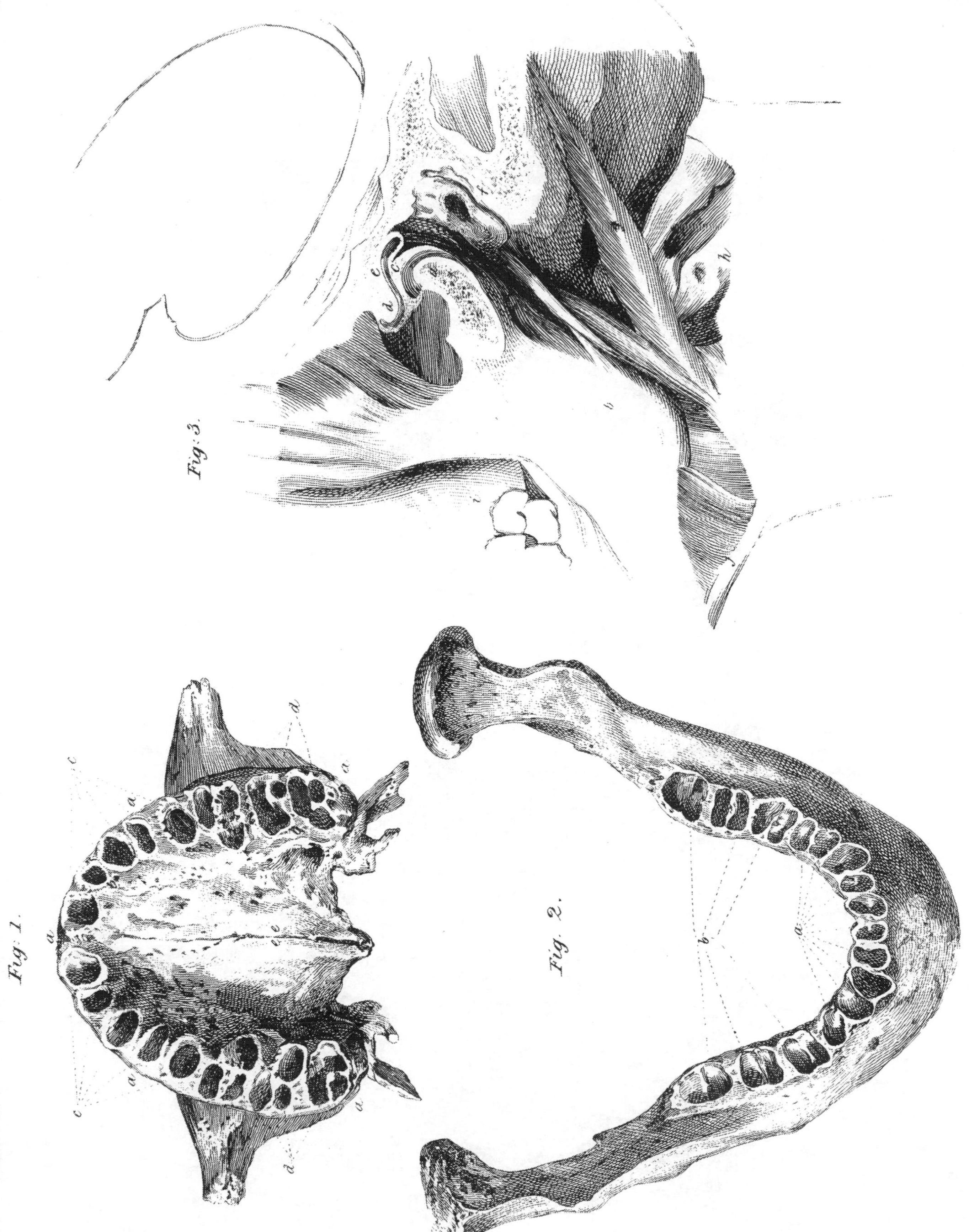

Fig. 3.

Fig. 1.

Fig. 2.

J. Basire. lithog.

PLATE II.

Fig: 2.

Fig. 1

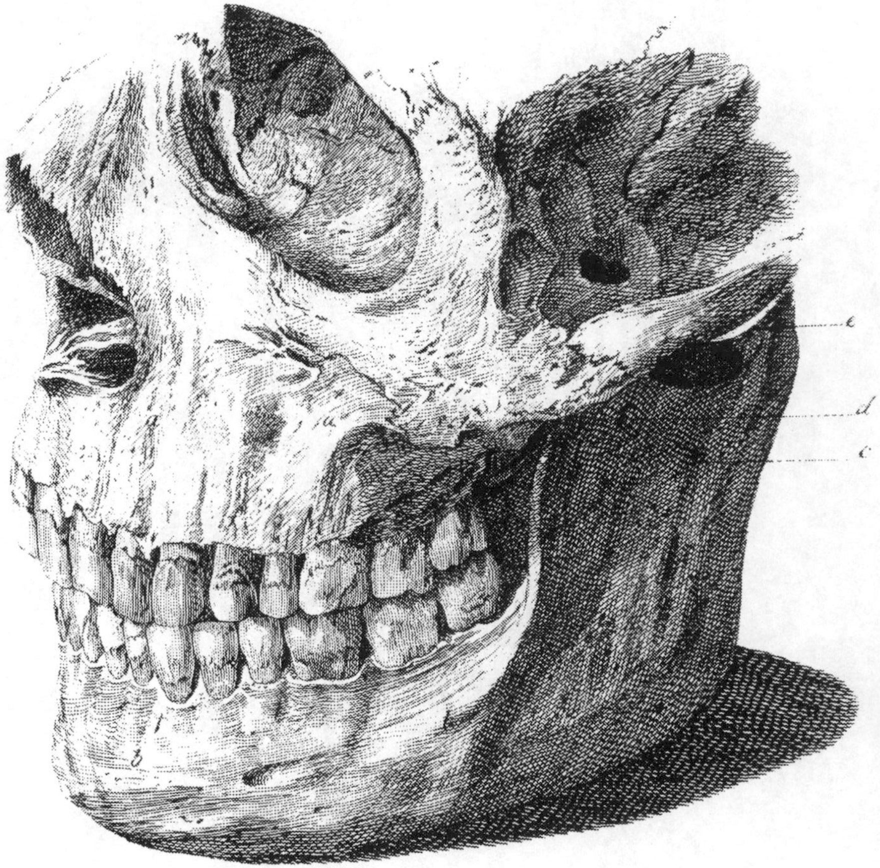

J. Basire, lithog.

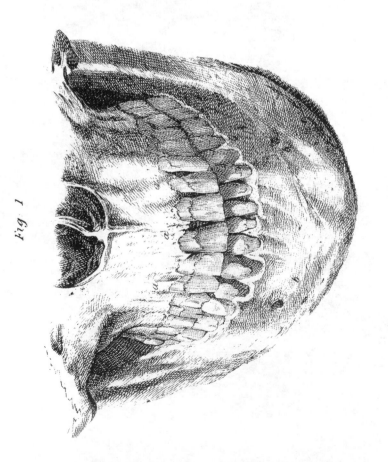

PLATE III.

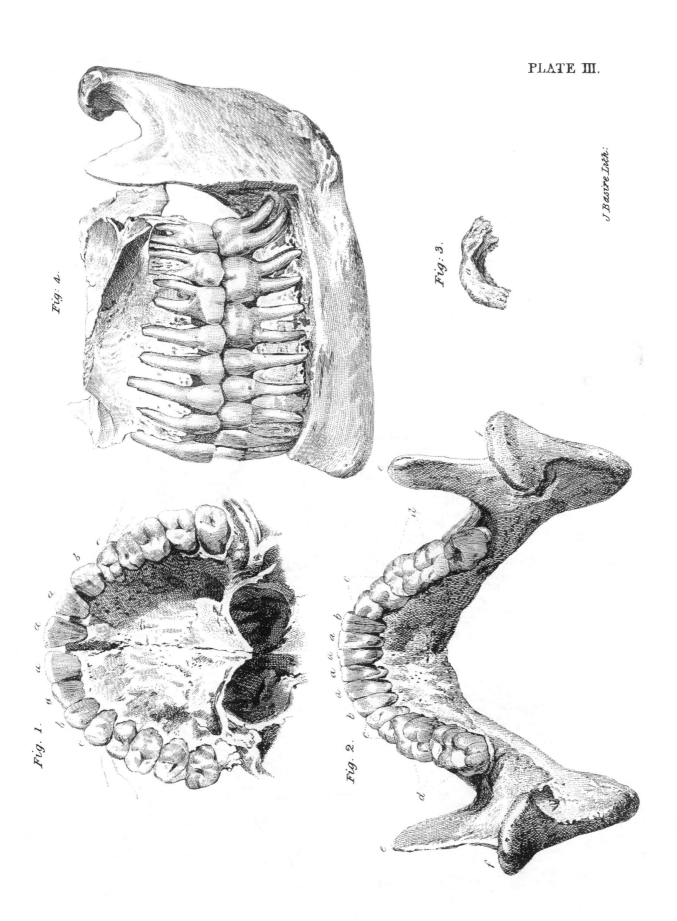

Fig: 4.

Fig: 3.

Fig. 1.

Fig. 2.

PLATE IV.

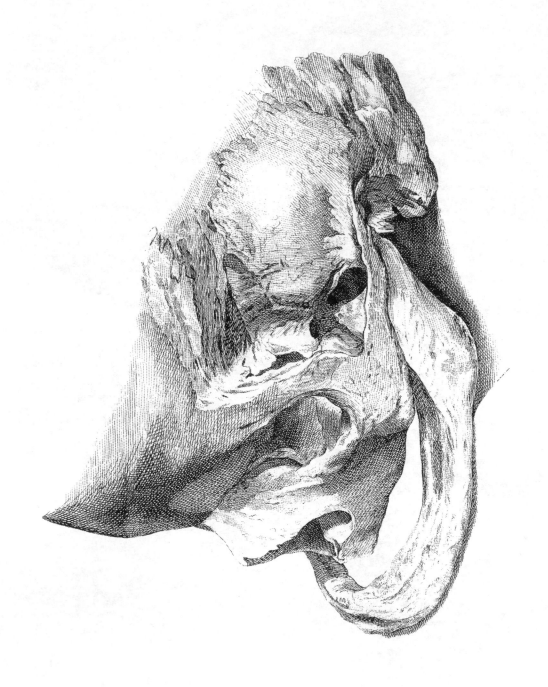

PLATE V.

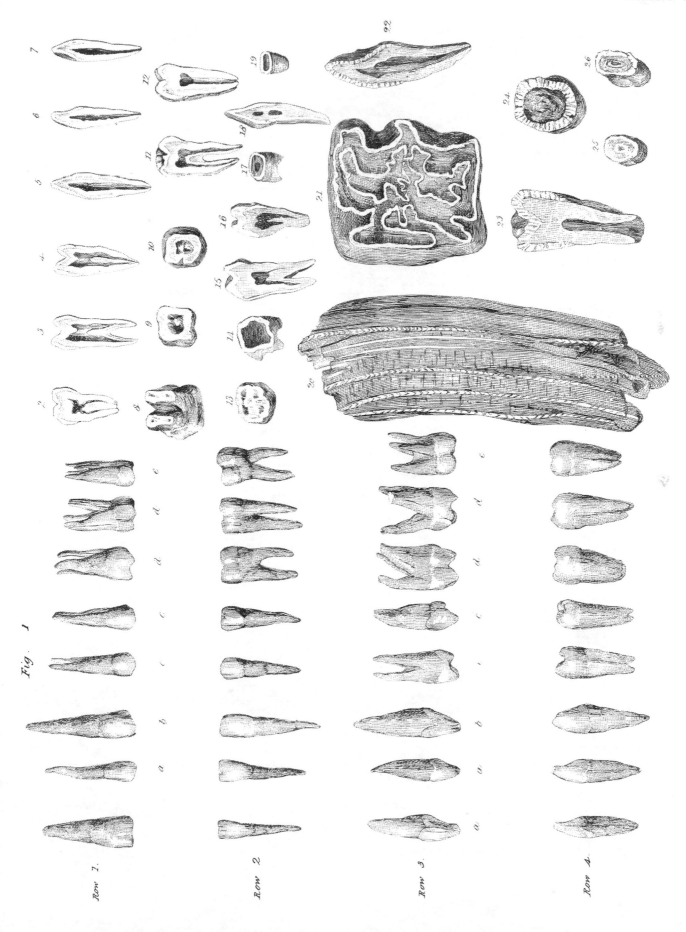

PLATE VI.

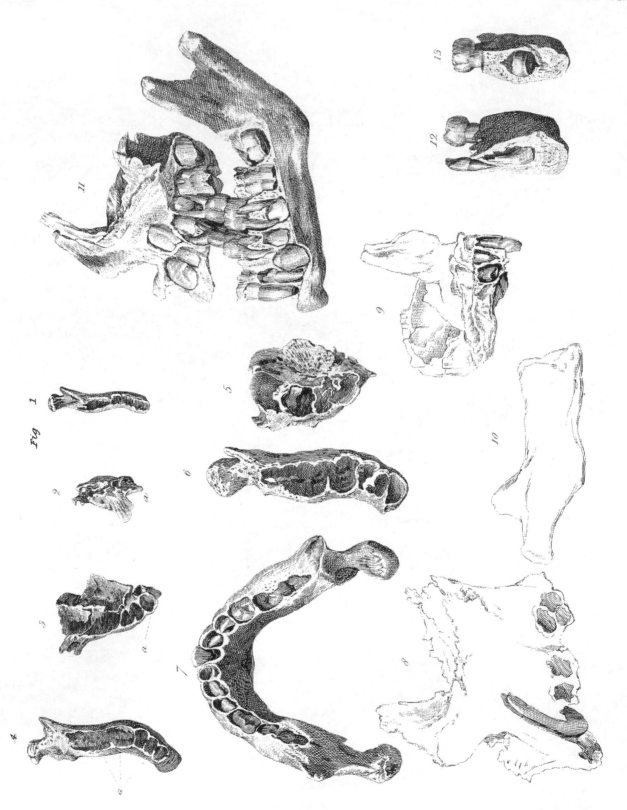

Fig 1

J. Green, litho.

PLATE VII.

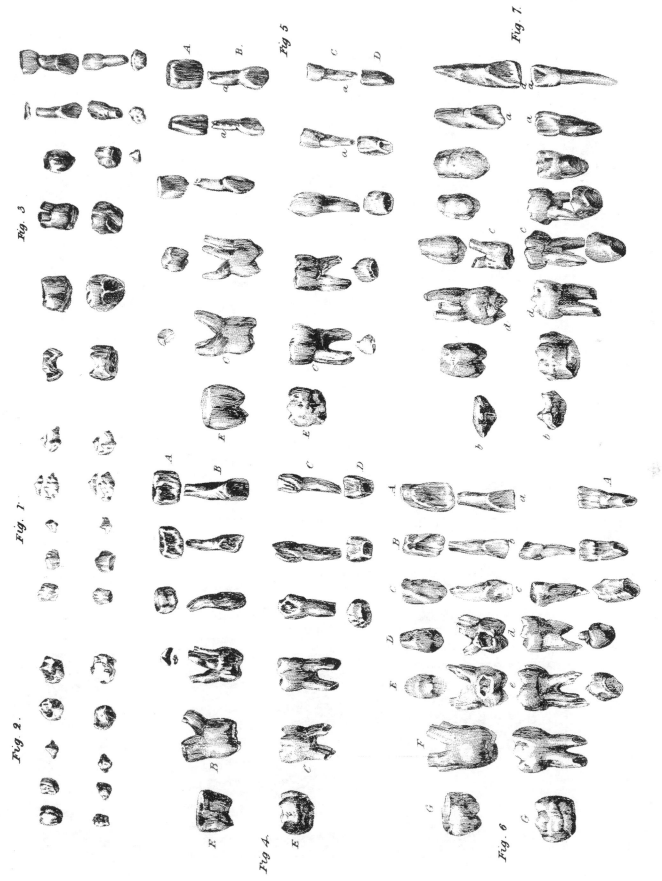

Fig. 1.

Fig. 5

Fig. 3.

Fig. 1.

Fig. 2.

Fig. 4.

Fig. 6.

J Basire lithog

PLATE VIII

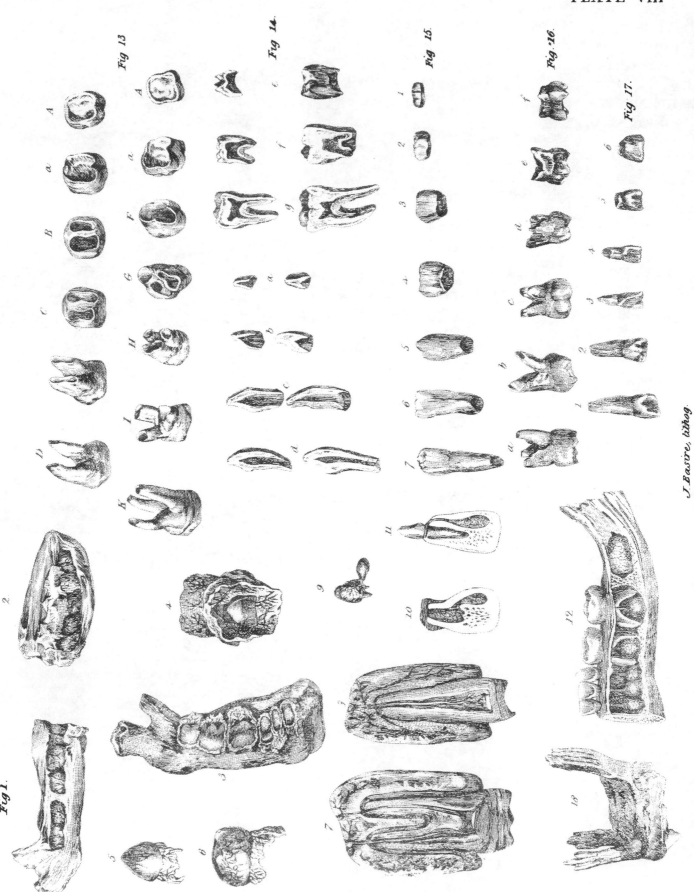

J. Basire, lithog.

Plate IX.

Fig. 1.

Fig. 2.

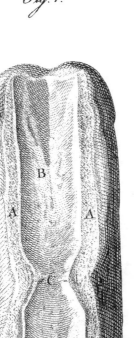

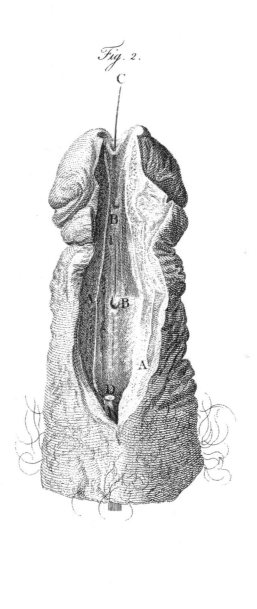

Wᵐ Bell del.

Wᵐ Sharp sc.

Plate X

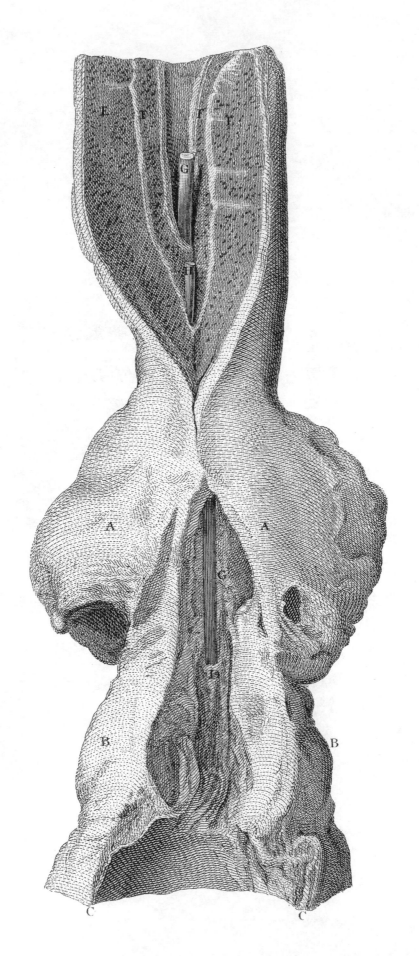

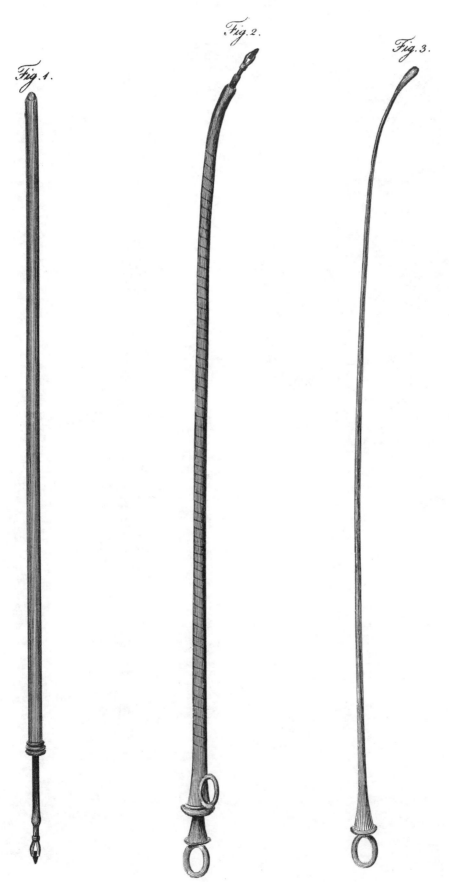

Plate.XI.

Fig.1.

Fig.2.

Fig.3.

Wᵐ Bell del.

Wᵐ Sharp sc.

Plate XII.

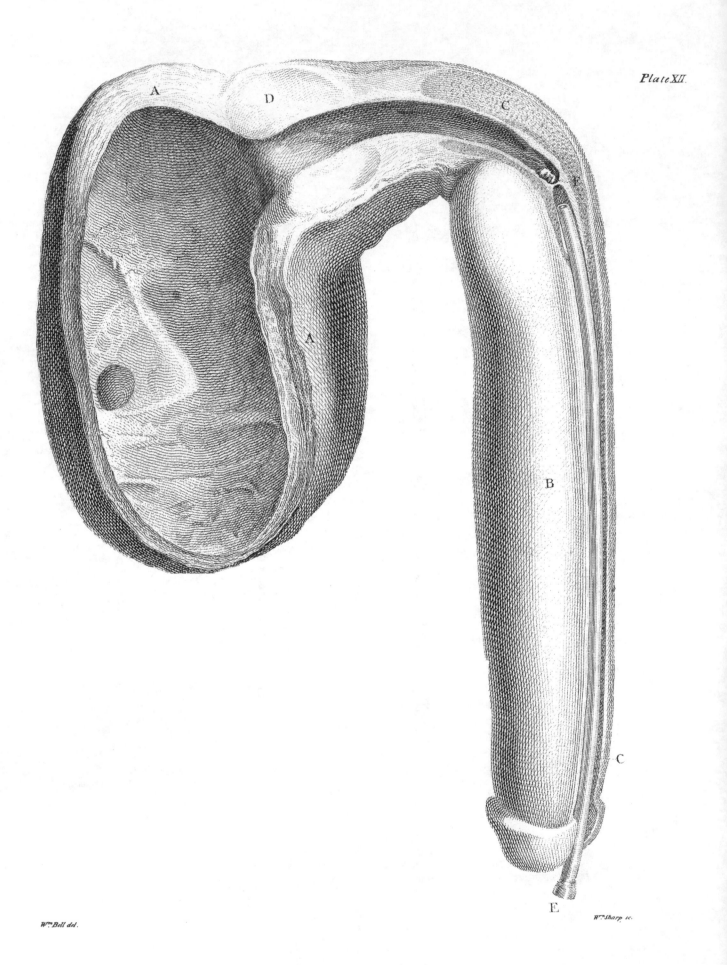

Plate XIII.

C

A

C
B

D

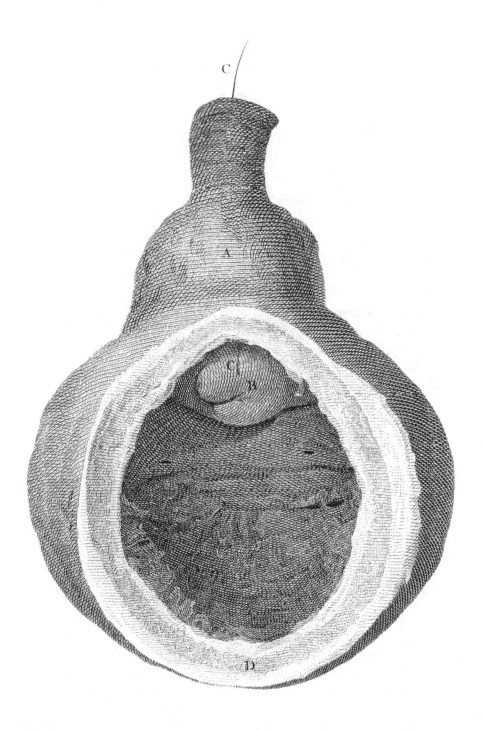

Wm Bell del.   Wm Sharp sc.

Plate XIV.

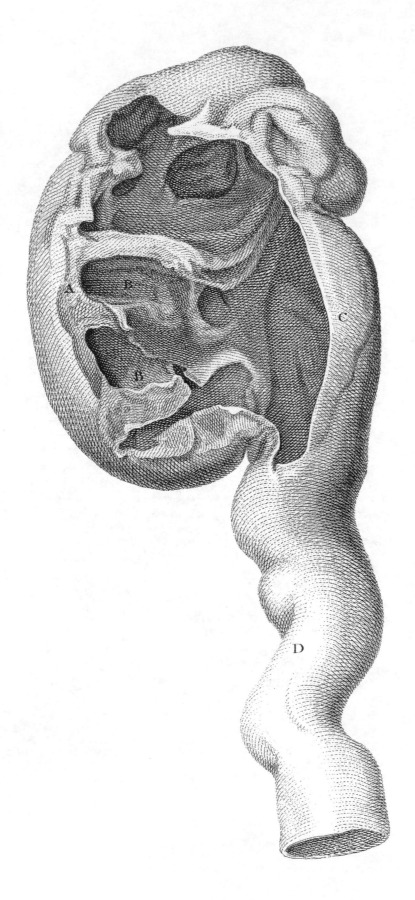

W^m. Bell del.

W^m. Sharp sc.

Plate XV.

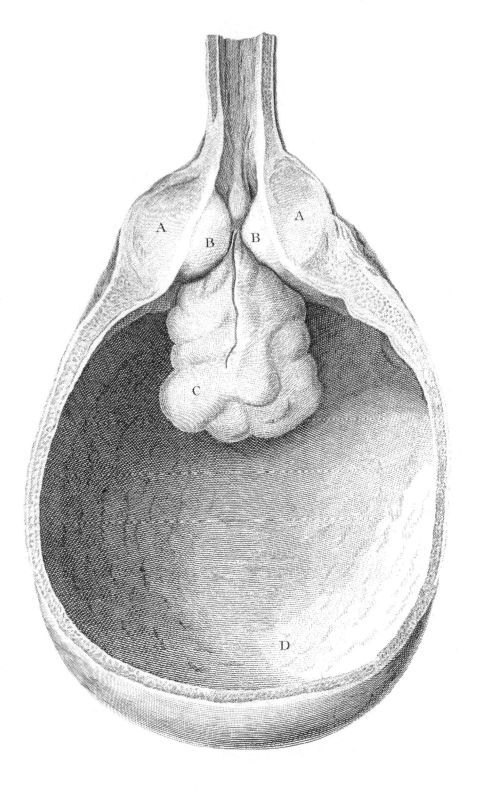

Plate XVI.

Fig. 1.

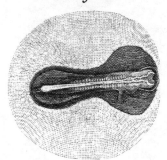

Fig. 2.

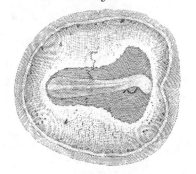

Fig. 3.

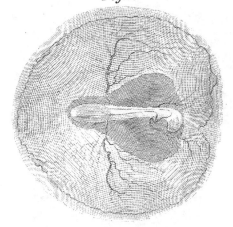

Plate XVII

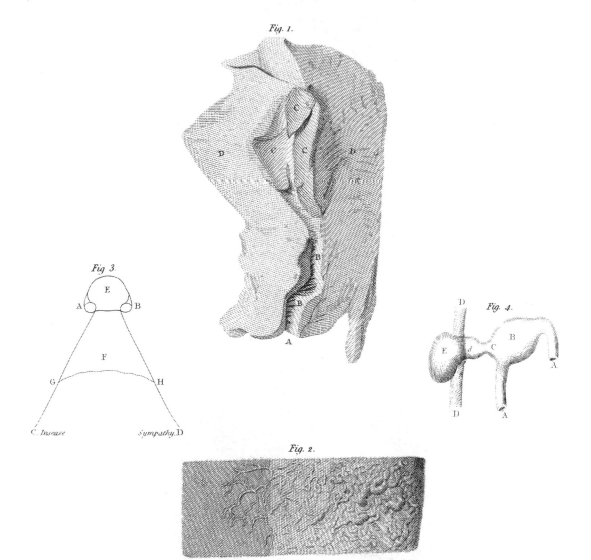

Fig. 1.

Fig. 3.

Fig. 4.

Fig. 2.

Plate.XVIII.

Fig. 2.

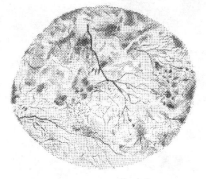

Fig. 1.

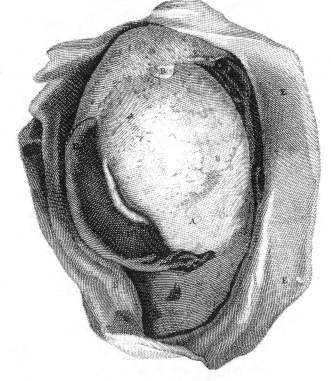

W. Bell del.

W. Skelton scalp.

Plate XIX.

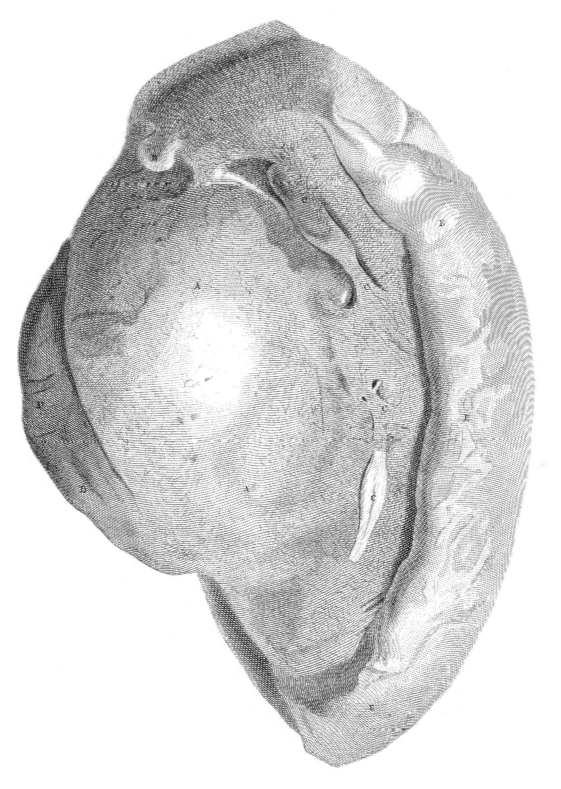

W. Bell del.

W. Skelton sculp.

Plate XX.

Fig. 3.

Fig 4

Fig. 1.

Fig. 2.

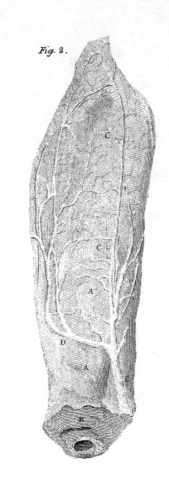

Fig 5.

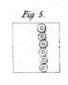

Fig 6.

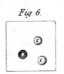

Fig 7

Fig. 8.

Fig 9.

Fig. 10.

W. Skelton sculp.

Plate XXI.

Fig.1.

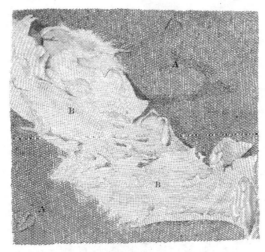

Fig. 3.

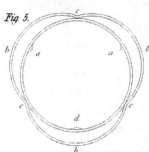

Fig 5.

Fig. 4.

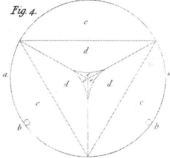

Fig.2.

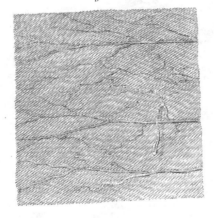

Fig. 6.

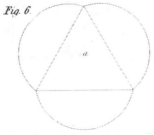

Plate XXII.

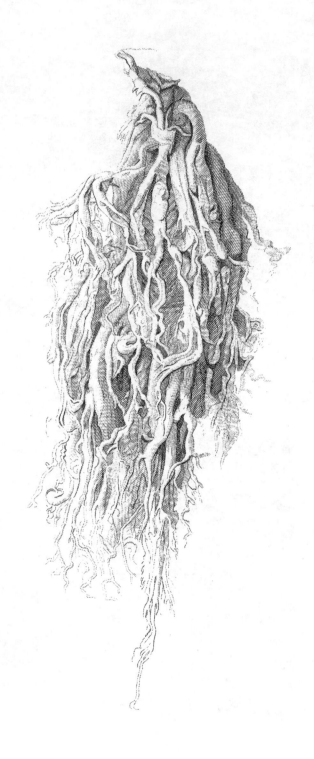

W. Skelton sculp.

Plate XXIII.

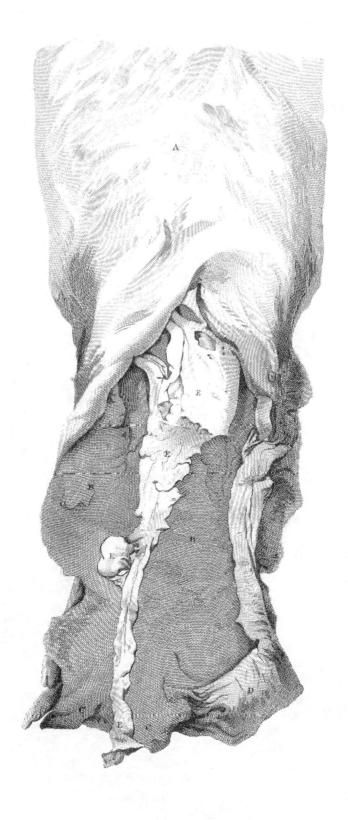

S.t Aubin del.

W. Skelton sculp.

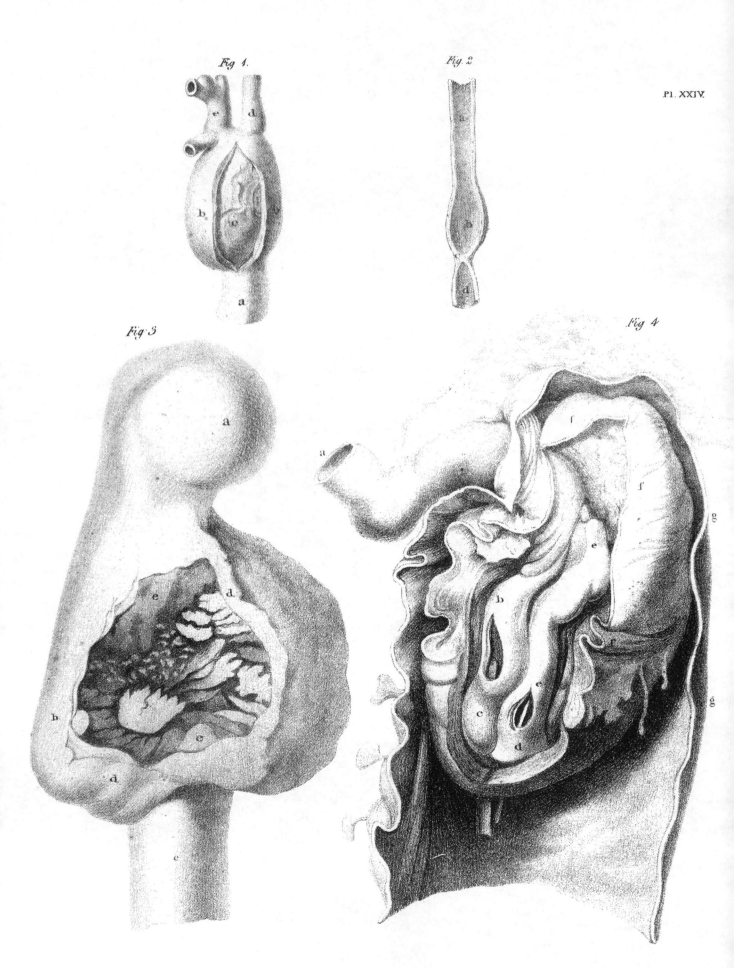

Pl. XXIV.

Fig. 1.

Fig. 2.

Fig. 3.

Fig. 4.

G. Scharf lithog.

Printed is. Baswt

Fig. 1

Pl. XXV.

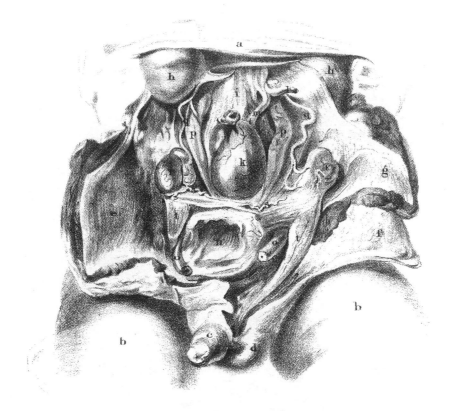

Fig. 2

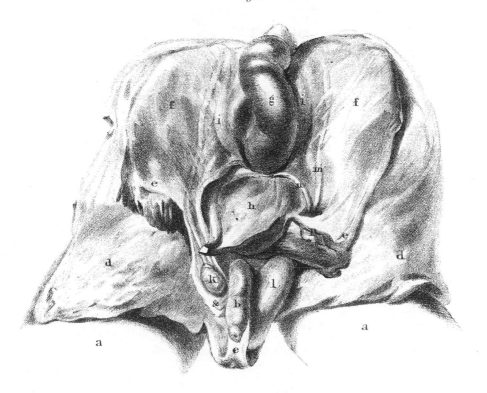

Pl. XXVI.

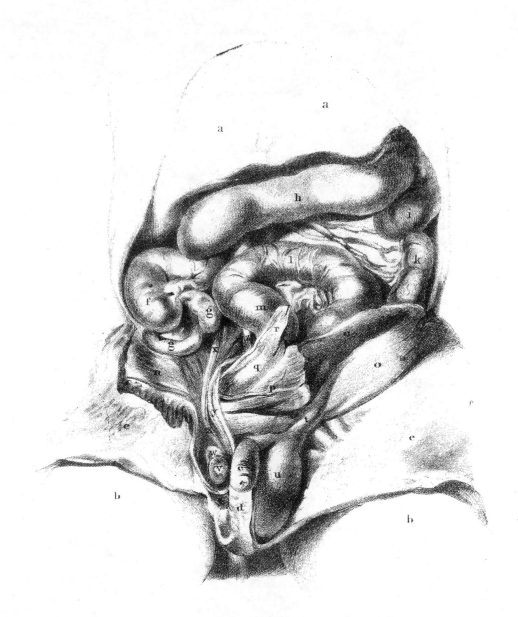

J.Van.Rymsdyk del. G.Scharf. lithog.

Printed by J.Basire.

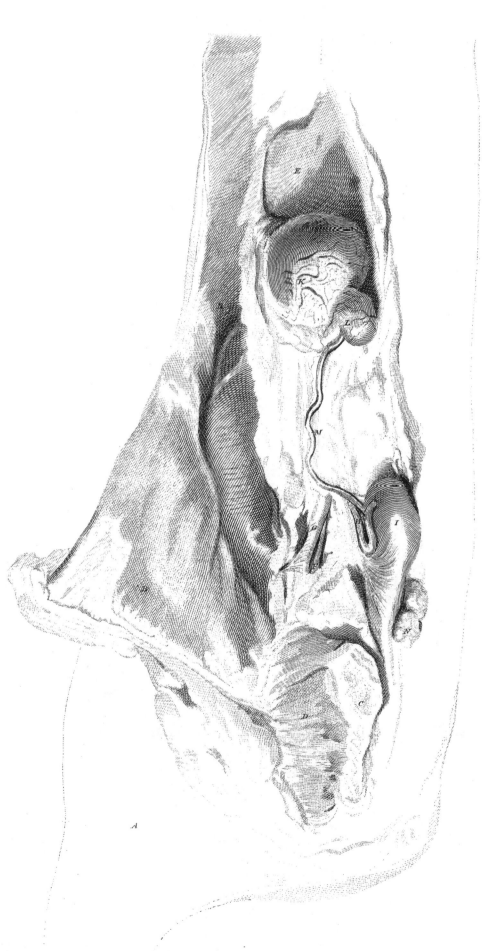

Plate XXVI.

J.V. Riemsdyk del.

W. Skelton sculp.

Plate XXVII.

Fig: I.

Fig: II.

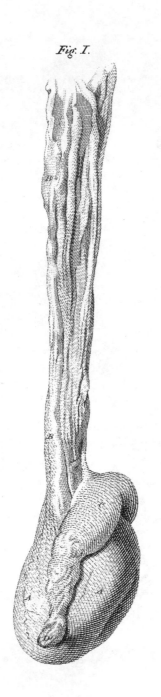

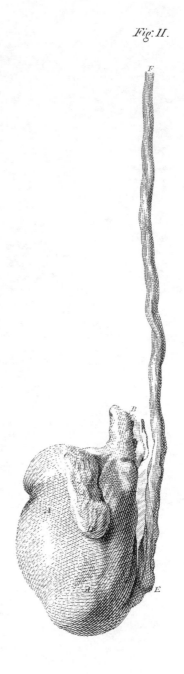

J.V.Riemsdyk del.

W.ᵐ Skelton sculp.

Plate XXVIII.

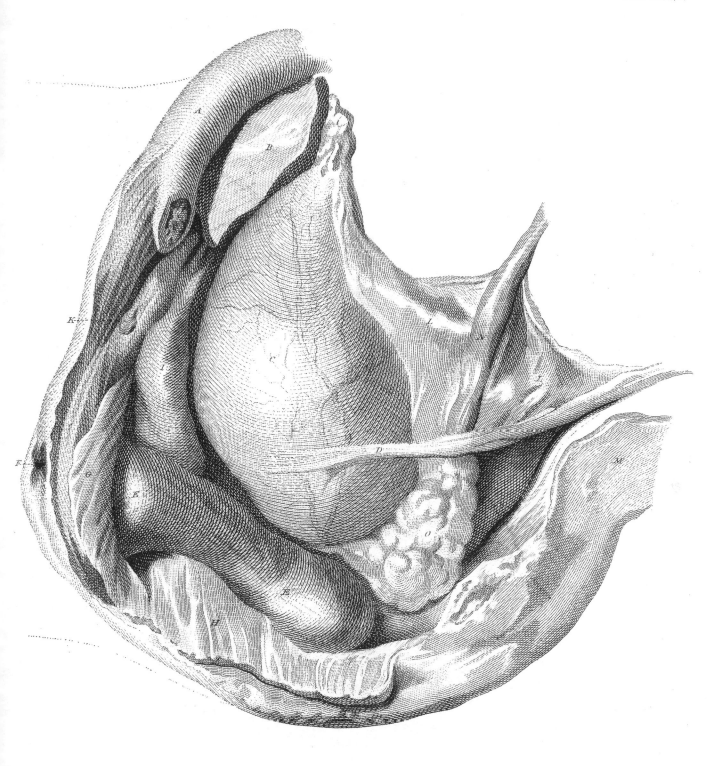

J. V. Riemsdyk del.

Wm. Skelton sculp.

Plate XXIX.

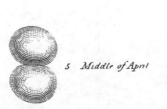

1 *January*

2 *Middle of February*

3 *Beginning of March*

4 *Latter end of March*

5 *Middle of April*

Plate XXX.

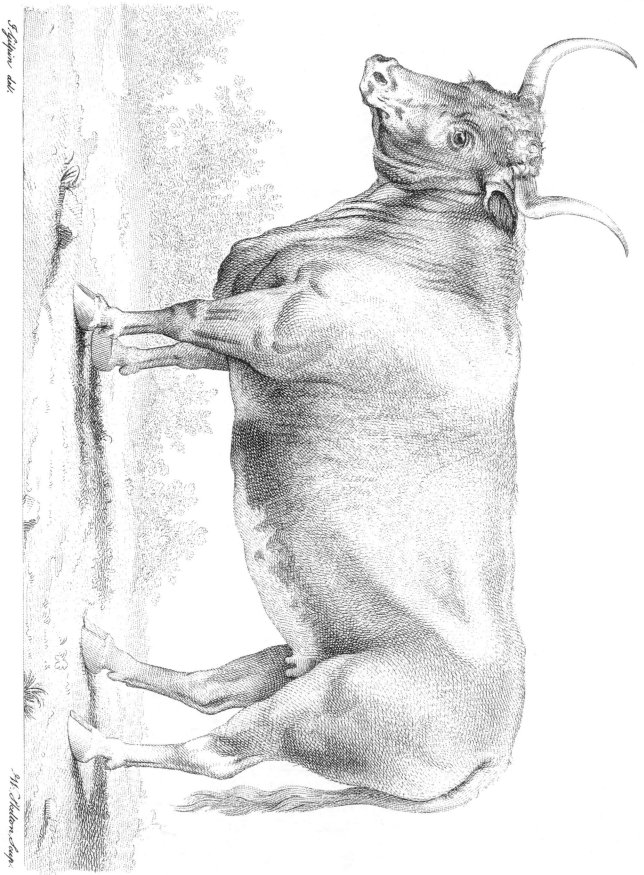

S.Gilpin delt.

W. Skelton Sculp.

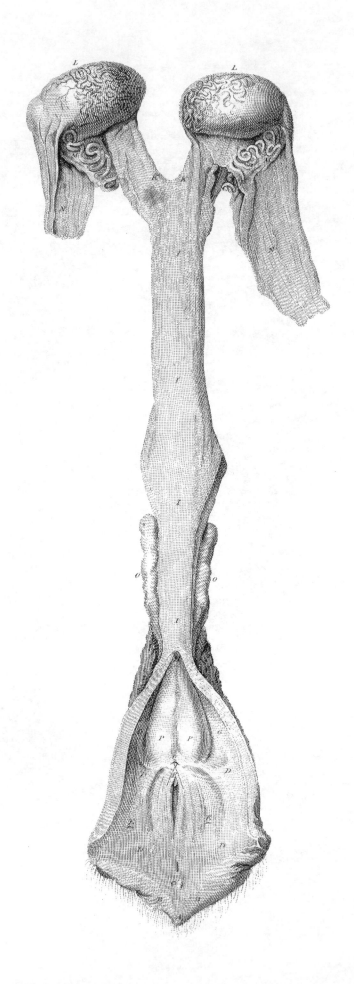

Plate XXXI

Plate XXXII

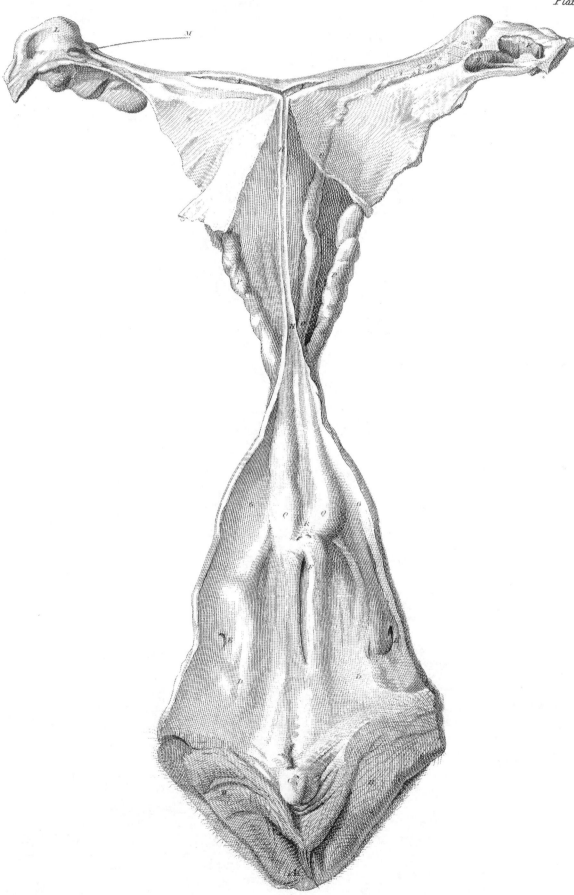

Wm Bell del.

Wm Skelton sculp.

Plate XXXIII.

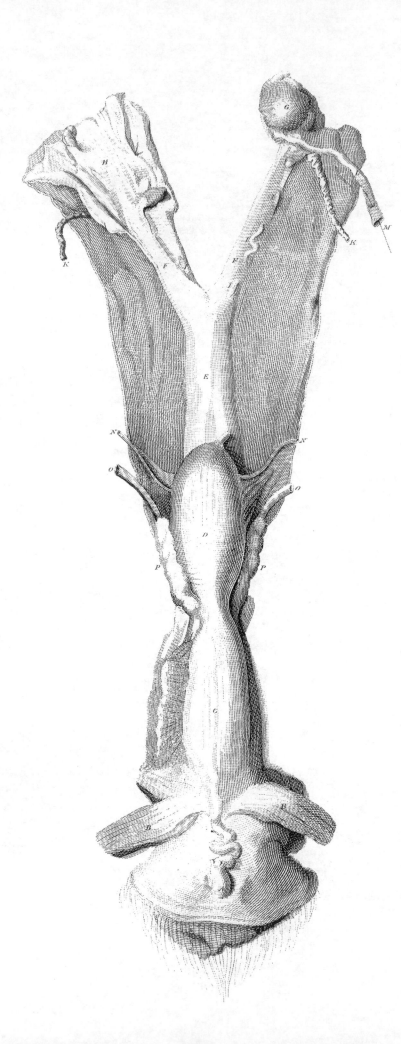

Wm Bell del.

Wm Skelton sculp.

Plate XXXIV

Fig. 1.

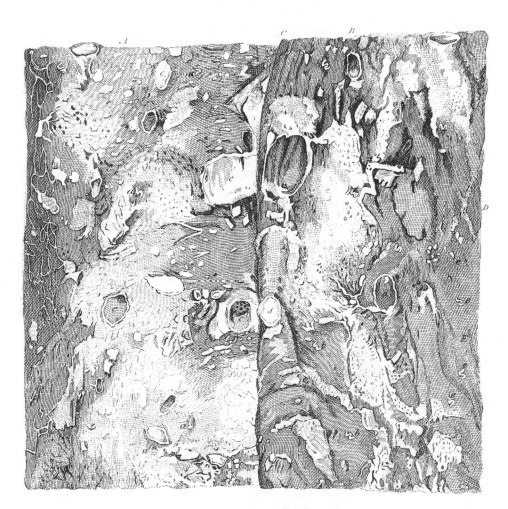

Fig 2

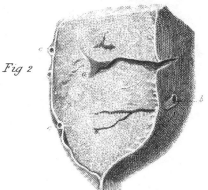

Wm Bell del.

Wm Skelton sculp.

Plate XXXV.
*Philos.Trans.*MDCCCXXII.*Plate XLIV.p.406.*

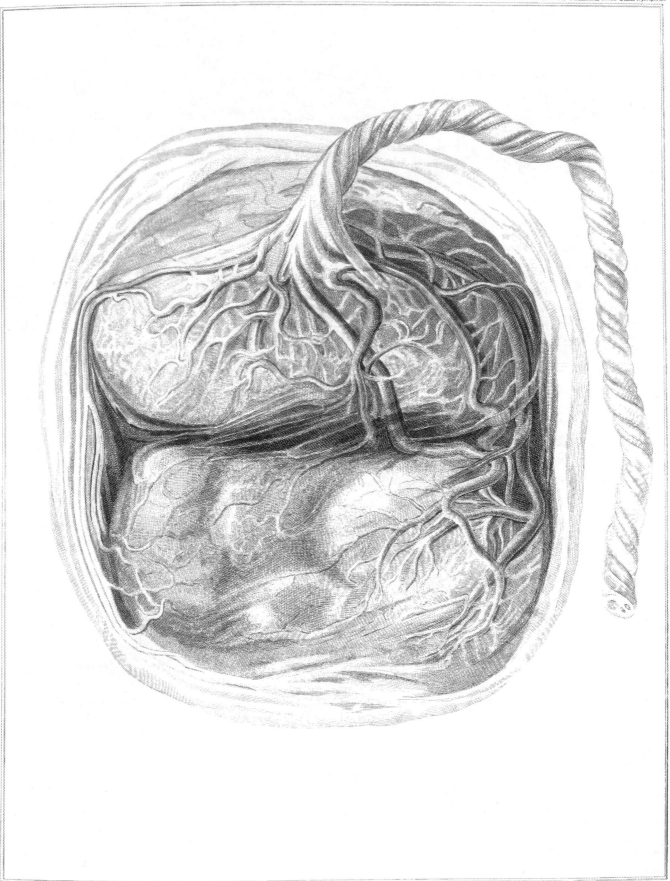

W. Clift del.   J. Basire sculp.

Plate XXXVI
Philos. Trans. MDCCCXXII. *Plate XLIV. p. 406.*

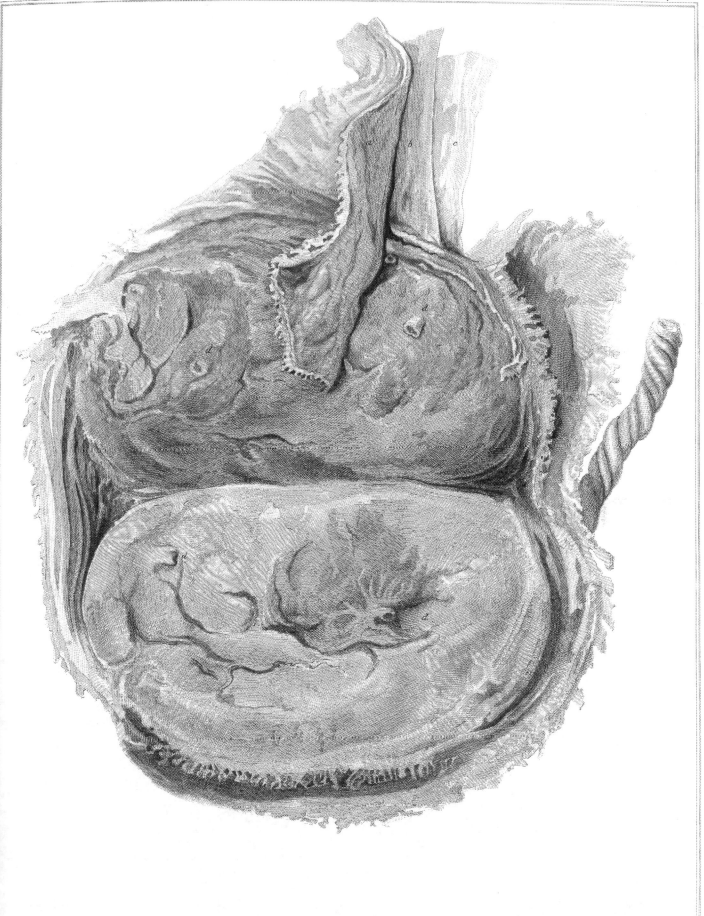

Plate XXXVII.

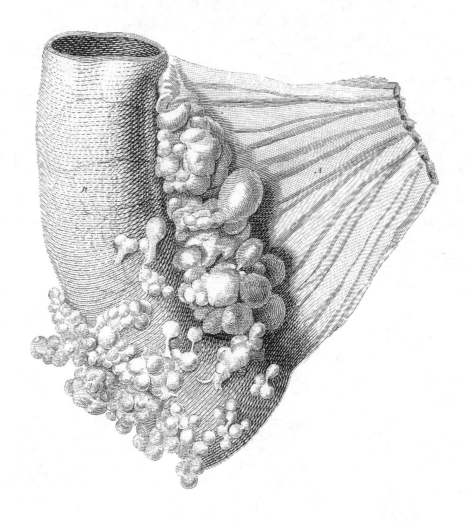

Plate XXXVIII.

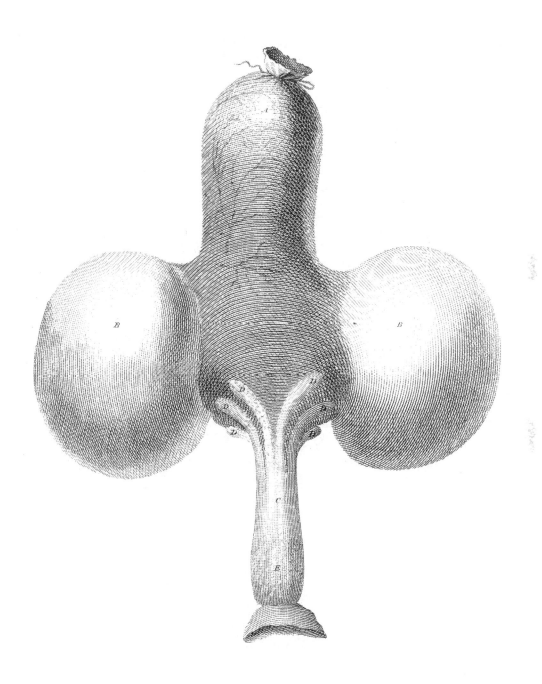

W.ᵐ Bell del.

W.ᵐ Skelton sculp.

Plate XXXIX.

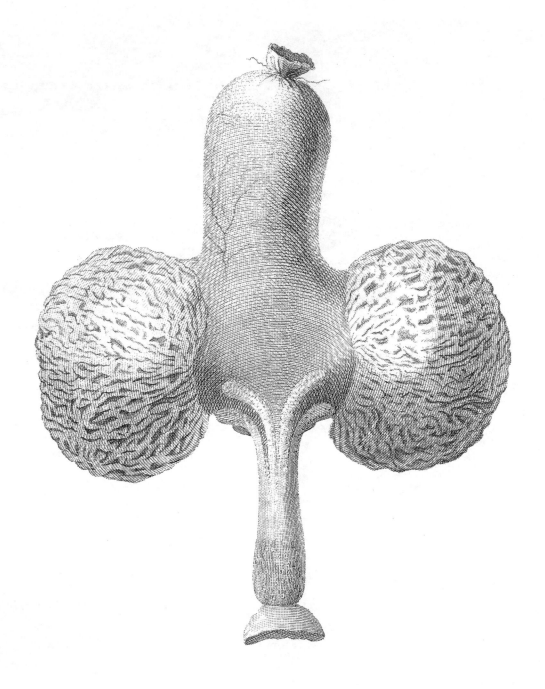

Plate XL.

Fig: I.

Fig: II.

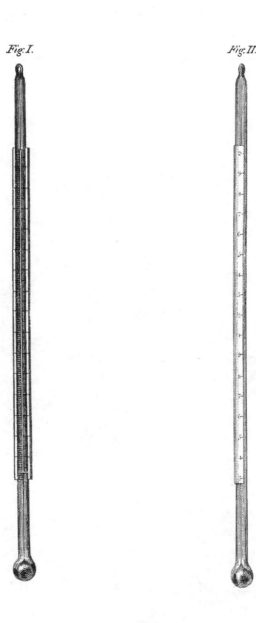

Plate XLI.

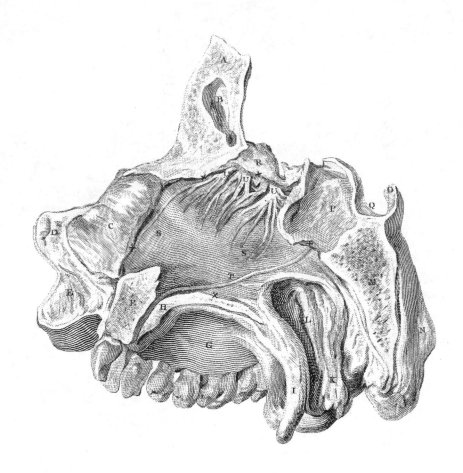

Plate XLII.

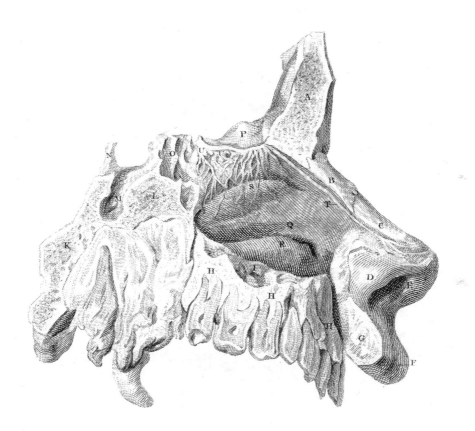

J. V. Reimsdyk del

W. Sharp sculp.

Fig. 1.

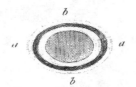

Fig. 2.

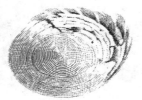

Plate XLIV.

Bayere Sc.

Phocœna. Orca.

Bell. d.

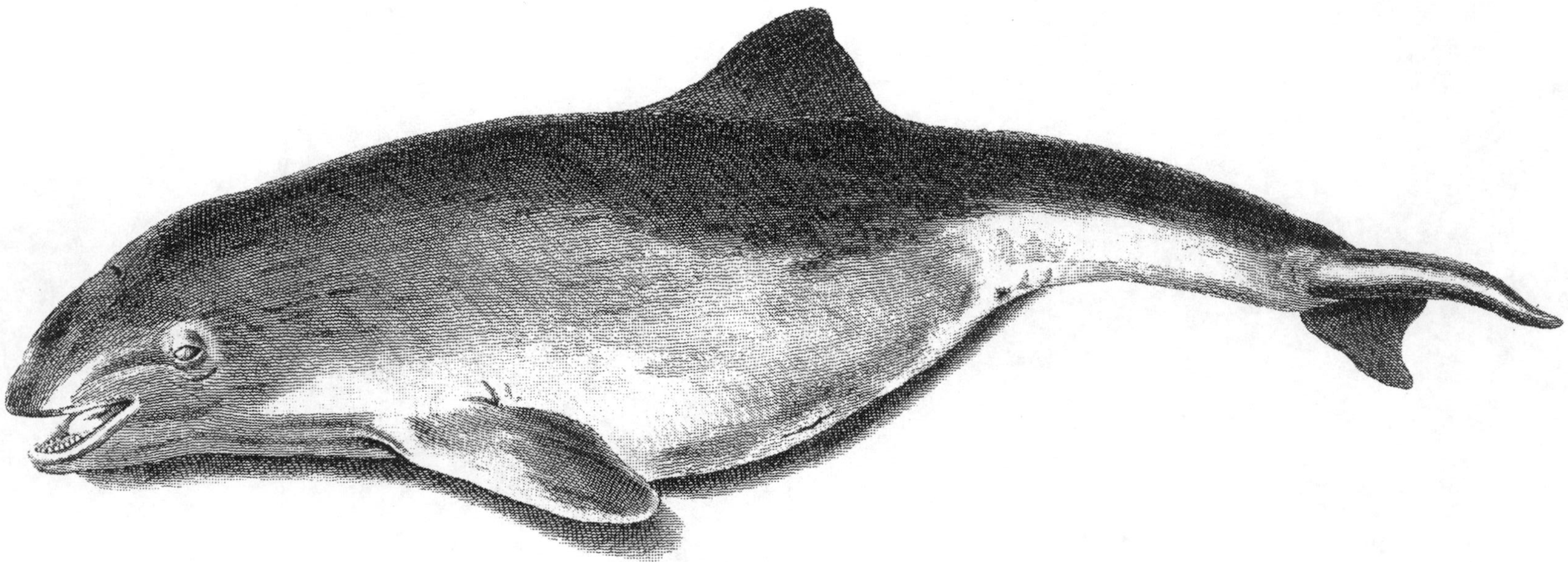

Plate XLV.

Philos. Trans. Vol. LXXVII. Tab. XVII. p. 450.

Phocæna communis.

Bell d.

Bayer Sc.

Plate XLVI.

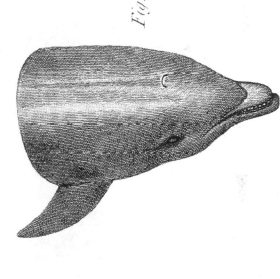

Fig. 1.

Fig. 2

Delphinus Tursio.

Plate XLVII

Philos. Trans. Vol. LXXVII. Tab. XIX. p. 460.

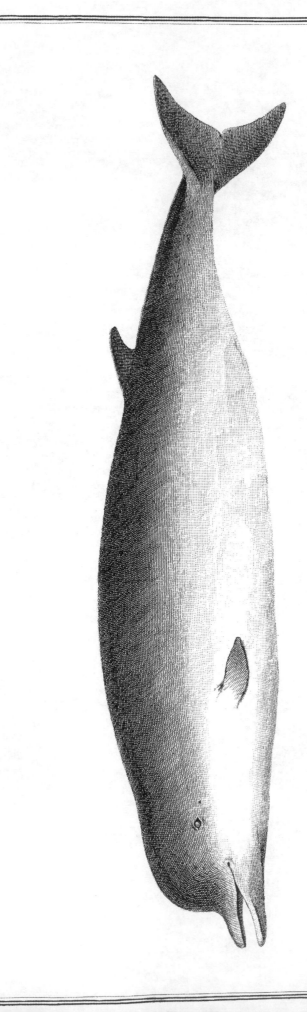

Hyperoodon bidens.

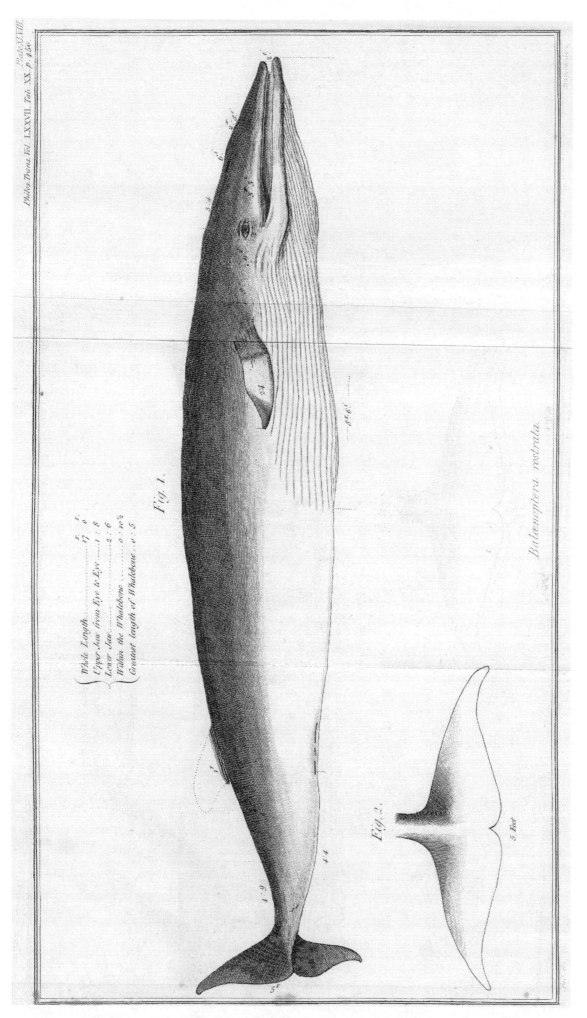

Fig. 1.

Whole Length		17 : 0
Upper Jaw from Eye to Eye		1 : 8
Lower Jaw		2 : 6
Within the Whalebone		0 : 10½
Greatest length of Whalebone		0 : 5

Fig. 2.

5 feet

Balænoptera rostrata.

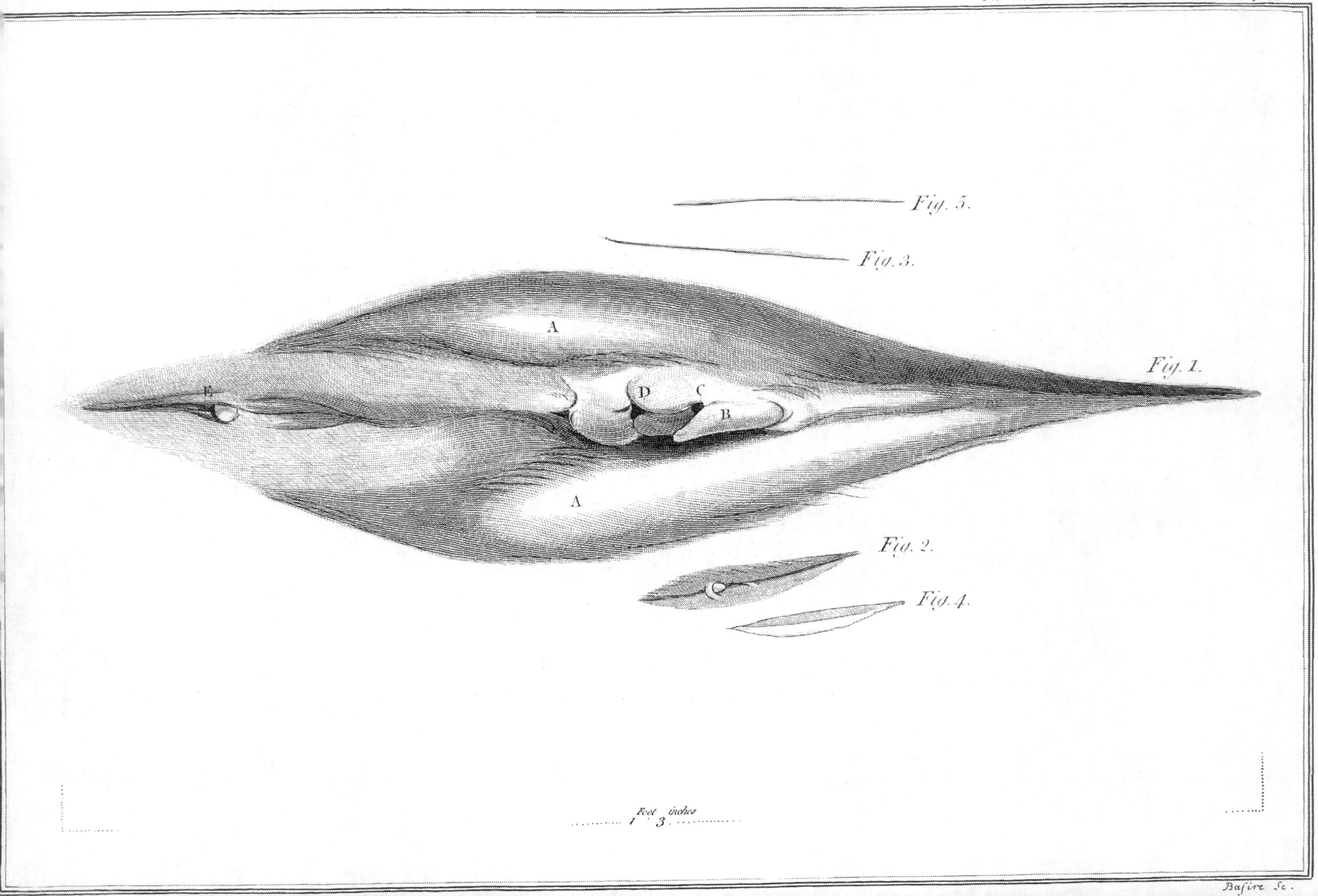
Fig. 5.
Fig. 3.
A
Fig. 1.
E
D
C
B
A
Fig. 2.
Fig. 4.
Foot inches
1 3

Basire Sc.

Plate L.
Philos. Trans. Vol. LXXVII. Tab. XXII. p 450

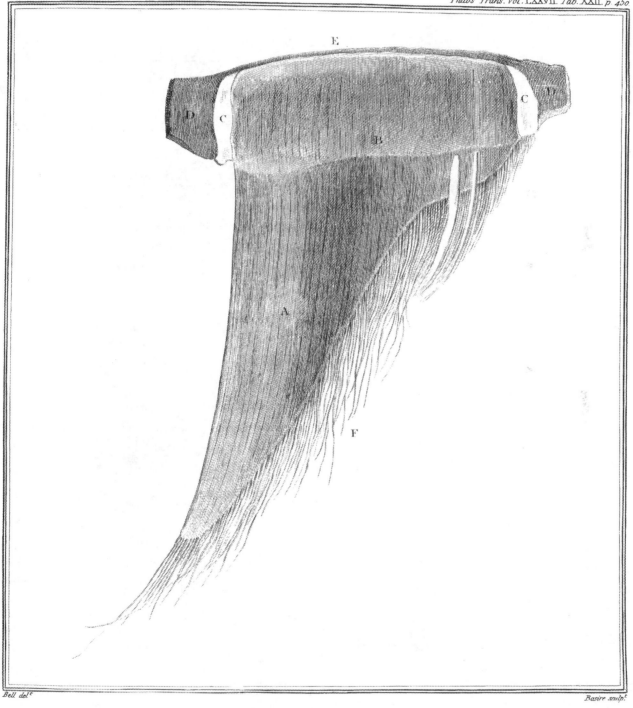

Plate LI.
Phil. Trans. Vol.LXXVII. Tab XXIII. p.450.

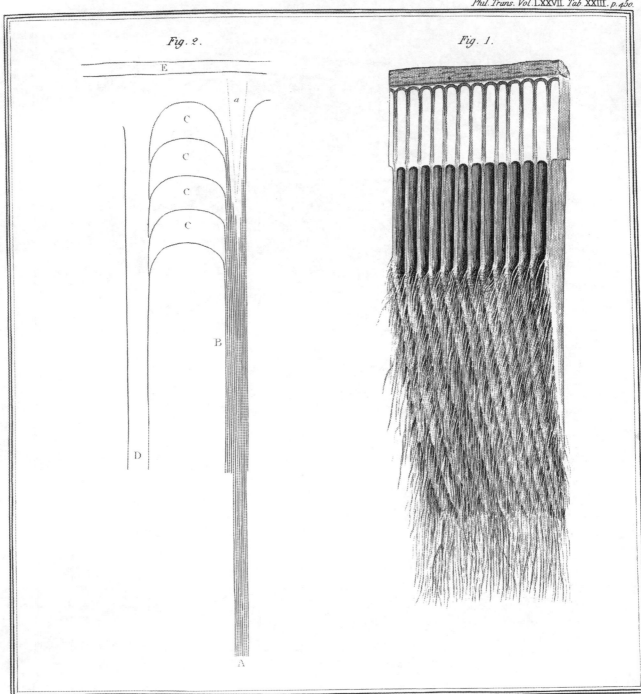

Fig. 2.

Fig. 1.

Bell delt.

Basire sculpt.

SIREN of Linnæus or Mud Iquana from S. Carolina

Plate 53

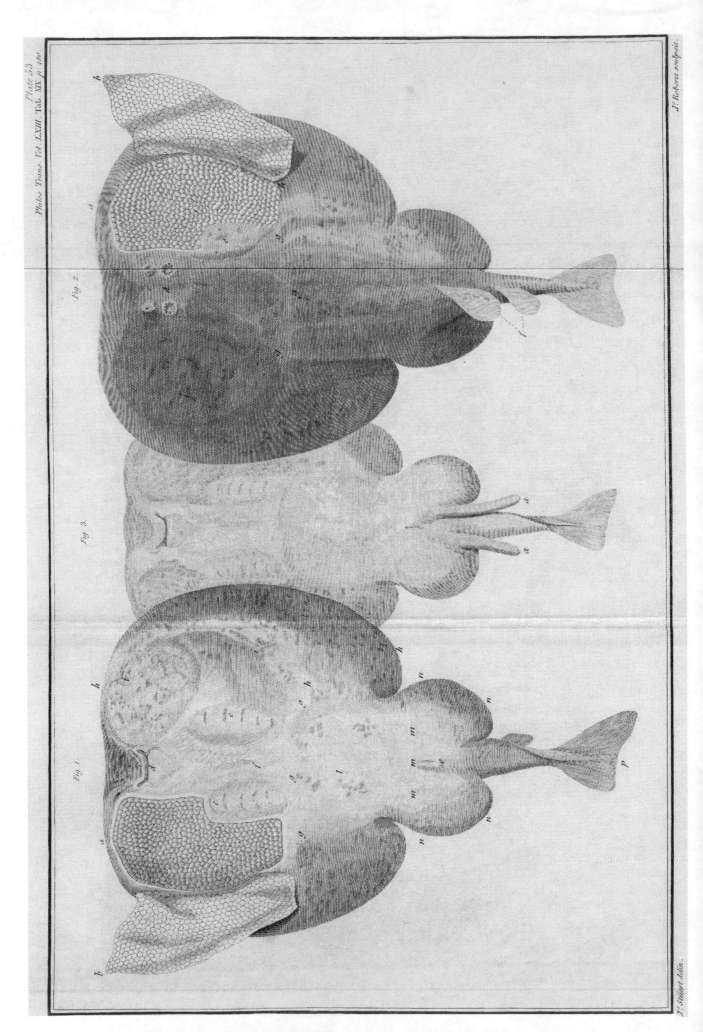

J. Roberts sculpsit.

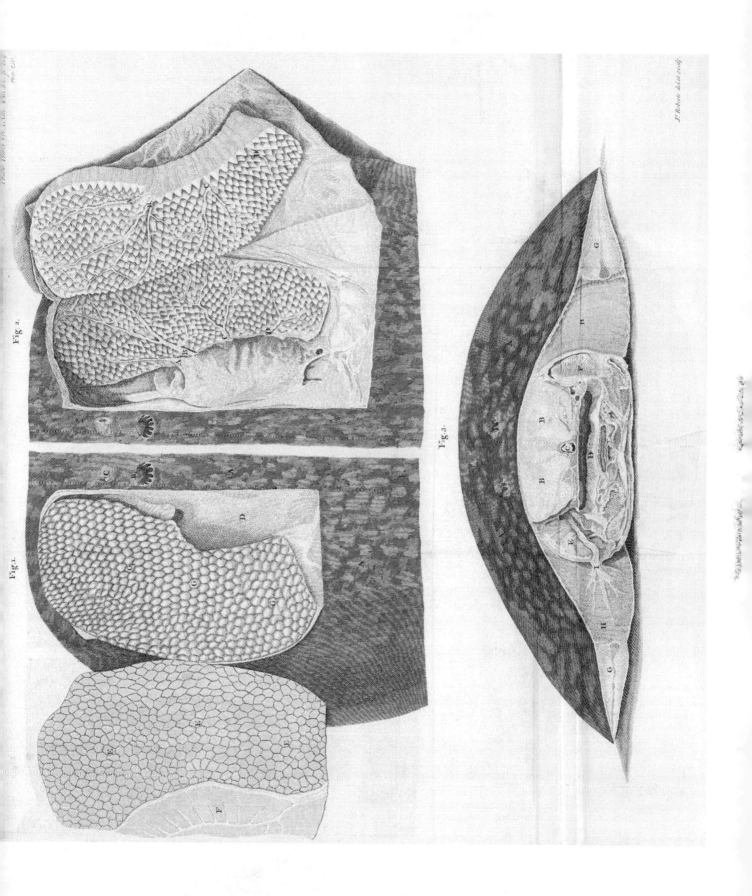

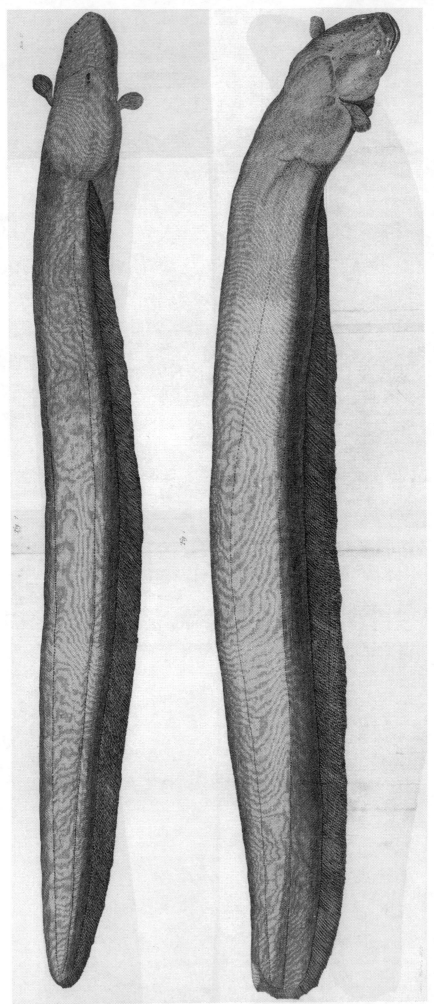

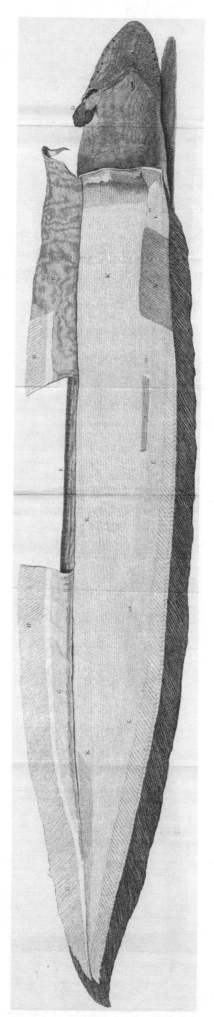

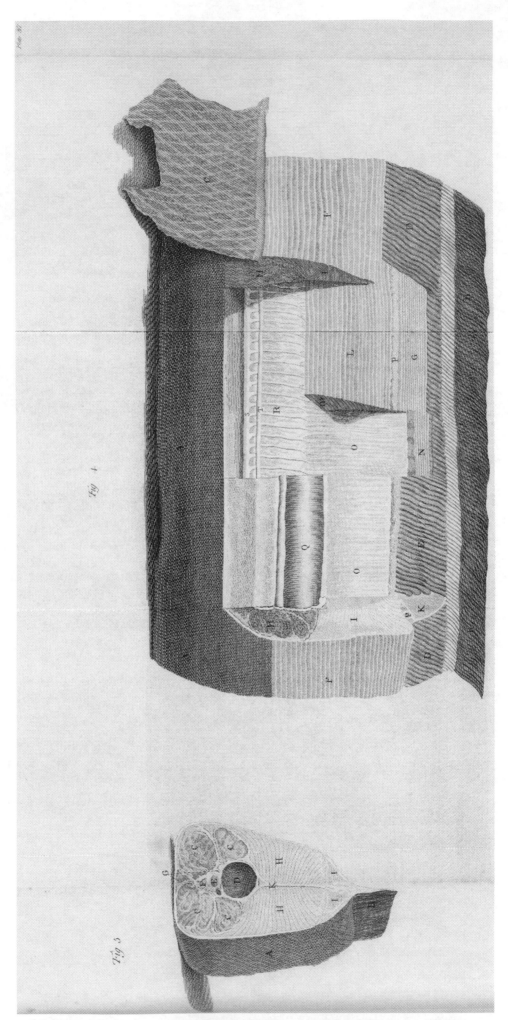

Philos.Trans.Vol. **LXXV.** *Tab.* **XI** *p.344.*
Plate LVIII.

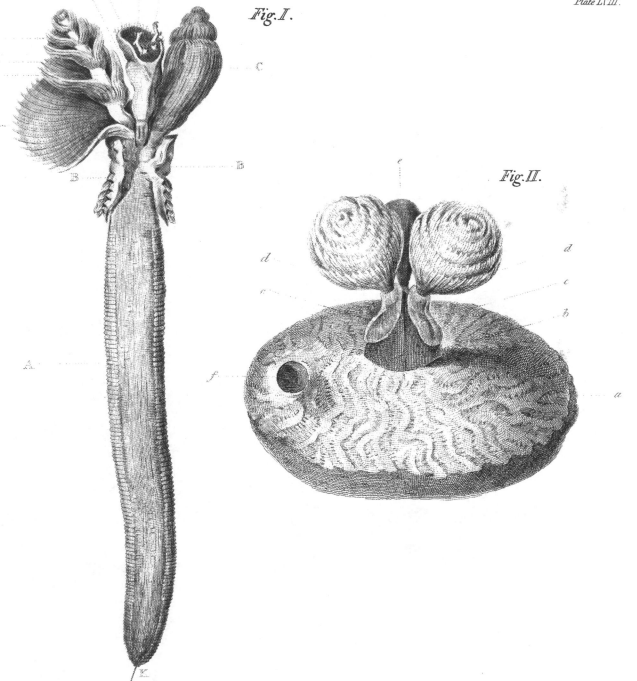

Fig.I.

Fig.II.

Basire sc

Philos. Trans. MDCCXCIV. Tab. XIX. p. 46.
Plate LIX.

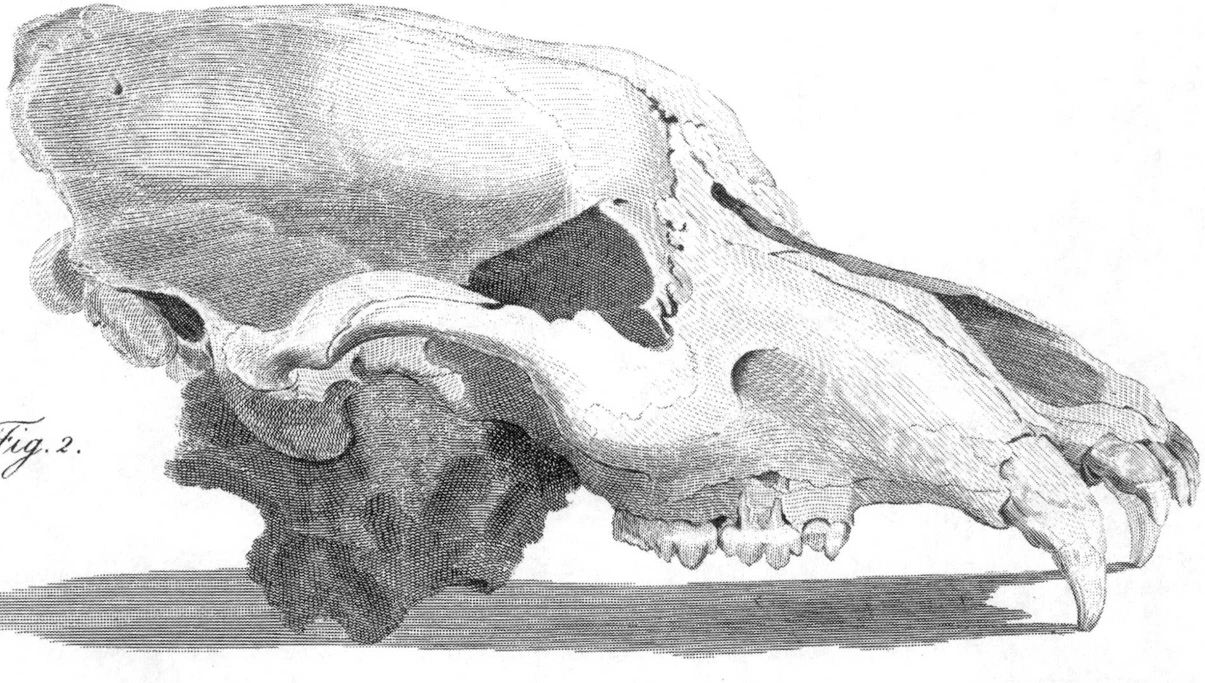

Basire Sc.

Fig. 1.

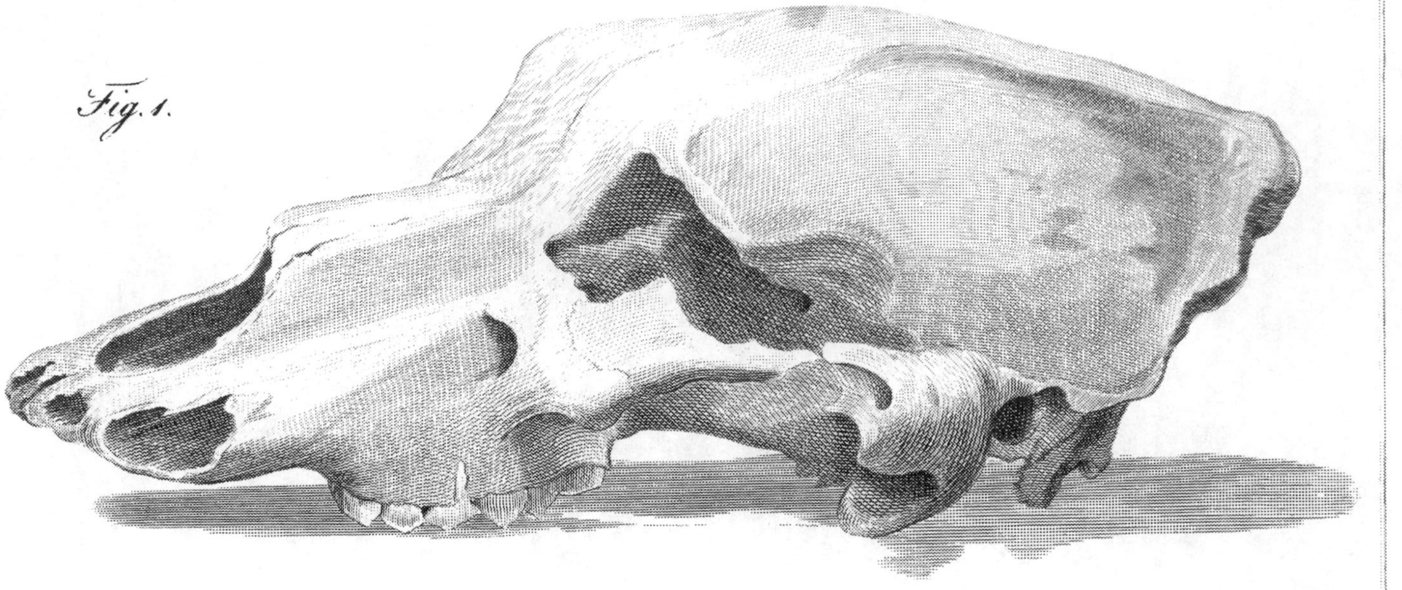

Fig. 2.

Fig.1.

Fig. 2.

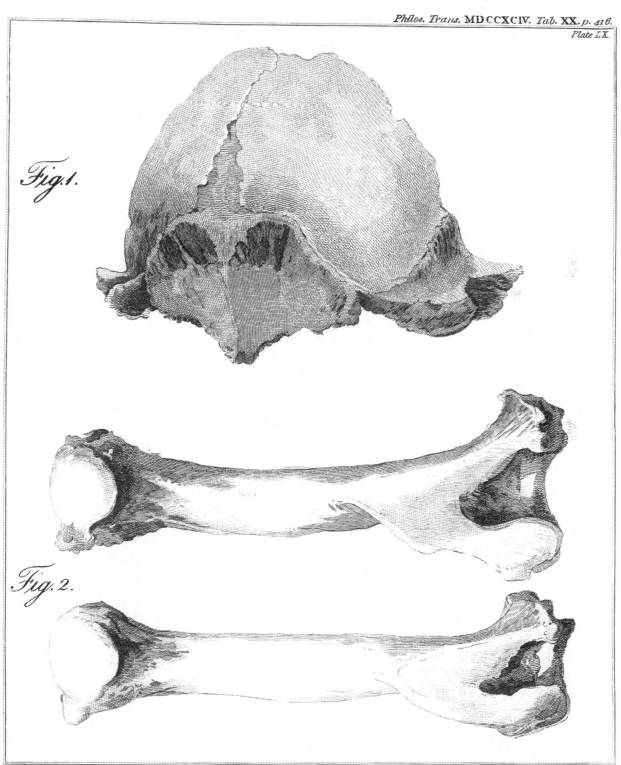

Basire. Sc.